Asclepius

the God of Medicine

Gerald D Hart MD

With editing of classical content and translation
of quotations by Martin Forrest PhD

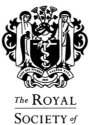

To Mervin and Win
with best wishes
Gerald
viii/MM

D1423834

The ROYAL
SOCIETY *of*
MEDICINE
PRESS *Limited*

1 Wimpole Street, London W1M 8AE, UK
207 E Westminster Road, Lake Forest, IL 60045, USA
http://www.roysocmed.ac.uk

British Library Cataloguing in Publication Data
A catalogue record for this book is available from the British Library

ISBN 1-85315-409-1

Typeset by Dobbie Typesetting Limited, Tavistock, Devon
Printed in Great Britain by Henry Ling Ltd, the Dorset Press, Dorchester, Dorset

Pio

et

Lio

'Asclepius, the son of Apollo and Coronis, learned many things from his father relating to the art of medicine. In addition, he discovered the art of surgery, the preparation of drugs and the power of roots as medicines. In general, he developed the art to such a degree that he was honoured as its leader and founder.'

Diodorus, *Bibliotheca historica*, V, 74, 6 (ET 355)

Contents

Acknowledgements

Special thanks are expressed to the following: Mrs Jacki Cyphery (Muskoka) for typing the initial draft; Michael and Nancy Hart (Toronto, Canada) for initial computer advice and launching me on the 'Information Highway' and Mr Dave Saddington (Dorchester, England) for on-going computer assistance and for keeping me on the road; Mr Richard Brickstock (Department of Classics, University of Durham), Dr Bruce Charles (retired) and Dr JTH Connor (formerly Hannah Institute for the History of Medicine, Toronto) for reading and commenting on the initial draft (1993); Dr Ann Woodward for editorial review on the second draft (1995); Ms Janet Illingworth-Cooper for editorial review of the third draft (1997); Professor Kate Ashcroft, Dean of the Faculty of Education, University of the West of England, Bristol for enabling Dr Martin Forrest to spend time working on the translations and text during 1998 and 1999; Mr Pat Horne (Toronto, Canada) for on-going encouragement and research assistance; and finally to Lilian Hart for reading innumerable drafts, encouragement and tolerance.

Grateful thanks are due to the following who assisted in correspondence, obtaining references, pictures and discussions: Mrs F Allen, London, England; Ms Lindsay Allison-Jones, Archaeological Museum Officer, Museum of Antiquities, Newcastle-upon-Tyne, England; Professor HJM Barnett, John P Robarts Research Institute, London, Ontario, Canada; Ms Jane Bircher, Keeper of Collections, Roman Baths Museum and Pump Room, Bath, England; Mr Richard Brickstock, Department of Classics, University of Durham, England; Dr Robin Birley, Vindolanda Trust, Bardon Hill, Northumberland, England; Dr Paul Bidwell, Principal Keeper (Archaeology), Arbeia Roman Fort and Museum, South Shields, England; Ms Nancy Bookidis, Assistant Director, Corinth Excavations, American School of Classical Studies, Athens, Greece; Ms Cindy Buhle, Bracebridge, Ontario, Canada; Dr P Carrington, Post Excavation Officer, Grosvenor Museum, Chester, England; Dr Bruce Charles, Associate Professor (retired), University of Toronto, Toronto, Canada; Ms Eve Cockburn, Paleopathology Association, Detroit, MI, USA; Dr JTH Connor, Toronto, Canada; Mr Derek J Content, Crow Hill, Houlton, Maine, USA; The Reverend Patrick Cotton, Parish Church of Saint John The Baptist, Tunstall, Lancashire, England; Professor D Cowan, Cancer Care Ontario, Toronto, Ontario; Dr EG Cross, Associate Professor, University of Toronto, Toronto, Canada; GE Dearlove, South Poorton, Dorset; the late Mrs Nina Drake, Toronto, Canada; Ms Julie Dalton, Communications Department, British Medical Association, London, England; Mrs Alison Harle Easson, Associate Curator in charge Greek and Roman Department, Royal Ontario Museum, Toronto, Canada; Professor Cesare Fieschi, Universita Degli Studi Di Roma-La Sapienza, Rome, Italy; Miss J Freeman, Department of Prehistoric and Romano-British Antiquities, The British Museum, London, England; Dr Denis Gibbs, Appleford, Oxon, England; Miss Bernadette Gillow, Curator, Greenwich Borough Museum, London, England; Offices of the Greek National Tourist Board, Montreal and Toronto, Canada; Dr R Gerald Guest, Toronto, Canada; Dr DS Harling, Secretary, The Huddersfield Medical Society, Huddersfield, Yorkshire, England; Michael Harling, Huddersfield, Yorkshire, England; Mr and Mrs R Harding, Toronto, Ontario; Dr David Hart, London, Ontario; Richard Hazzard Esq, Toronto,

Canada; Dr Martin Henig, Institute of Archaeology, Oxford, England; Mrs Fiona Hepburn, Perthshire Tourist Board, Blairgowrie, Scotland; Mr Fraser Hunter, Department of Archaeology, National Museums of Scotland; Dr RPJ Jackson, Department of Prehistoric and Romano-British Antiquities, The British Museum, London, England; the late Br Flavian Keane, OH Ospedale Fatebenefratelli, Rome, Italy; Ms Janet Larkin, Department of Coins and Medals, The British Museum, London, England; John C Lavender, Classic Numismatic Group Inc, Lancaster, PA, USA; Professor J Lazenby, Department of Classics, University of Newcastle, England; Dr Elizabeth Lazenby, Department of Classics, University of Newcastle, England; Dr GAS Lloyd, Consultant Radiologist, The Royal National Throat, Nose and Ear Hospital, London, England; Dr CJM Martin, The Department of Scottish History, University of St Andrews, Scotland; Mr Paul McCullouch, Historic Resources Centre, Winchester, England; Eric J McFadden, Director Classic Numismatic Group Inc, London, England; Mr Peter Milligan, formerly at the Photographic Department, Toronto East General Hospital; the late Mr Enoch Myatt, Toronto, Canada; Professor GR Paterson, Executive Director (retired), Hannah Institute for the History of Medicine, Toronto, Canada; Mr RNR Peers, FSA, Curator (retired) Dorset County Museum, Dorchester, Dorset, England; Ms Georgina Plowright, Curator, English Heritage: Hadrian's Wall Museums and Department of Archaeology, The University, Newcastle-upon-Tyne, England; Mrs Felicity Pope, former Curator, The Canadian Museum of Health and Medicine at the Toronto Hospital, Toronto, Canada; Ms Gil Poulter, Department of Archaeology, Perth Museum and Art Gallery, Perth, Scotland; Mrs Gloria L Pratt, Gravenhurst, Ontario, Canada; Professor Paulo Rossini, Ospedale Fatebenefratelli, Rome, Italy; Mr D Robinson, Keeper of Archaeology, Grosvenor Museum, Chester, England; Mr Colin Richardson, Head of Archaeology, Carlisle Museums and Art Gallery, Carlisle, Cumbria, England; Mr RA Rutland, Keeper of Archaeology, Jewry Wall Museum, Leicester, England; Mrs Merry Ross, Dorchester, Dorset, England; Professor Robert Salter, The Hospital for Sick Children, Toronto, Canada; the late Dr Howard Savage, Department of Anthropology, University of Toronto, Toronto, Canada; Dr Grace Simpson, Curator, Chesters Museum, Hadrian's Wall, Northumberland, England; Dr Marja Soots, Toronto, Canada; Dr Bruce P Squires, Editor-in-Chief, Publications, Canadian Medical Association, Ottawa, Canada; Professor Ernie Steib, Associate Dean, Faculty of Pharmacy, University of Toronto, Canada; the late Professor WE Swinton, Massey College, University of Toronto, Toronto, Canada; Miss J Vale, Heritage Development Officer, County Hall, Maidstone, Kent, England; Ms Michelle Villeneuve, Queens University, Kingston, Ontario, Canada; Mr Kerry Wetterstrom, Classic Numismatic Group, Lancaster, PA, USA; Mr Ian Whan, formerly at the Photographic Department, Toronto East General Hospital; Dr RH White, Leverhulme Research Fellow, Field Archaeology Unit, University of Birmingham, Birmingham, England; Dr CH Wilkens, Toronto, Canada; Dr Ann Woodward, Research Fellow, University of Birmingham, Birmingham, England; and Professor Dr G Zinserling, Archaeologisches Institute, Universitat Jena, Germany.

The author and publisher gratefully acknowledge the following for providing and allowing reproduction of quotations and illustrations: The Johns Hopkins University Press, Baltimore, MD, US; Bulletin of the History of Medicine; The Trustees of the British Museum (Department of Coins and Medals, Department of Prehistoric and Romano-British Antiquities), London, England; American School of Classical Studies, Corinth Excavations, Athens, Greece; *British Medical Journal* and the British Medical Association, London, England; Bibliothèque Nationale de France, Service Photographique, Paris, France; Canadian Museum of Health and Medicine, Toronto, ON, Canada; Canadian

Medical Association and *Canadian Medical Association Journal*, Ottawa, ON, Canada; Dorset County Museum, Dorchester, England; Hoffman-La Roche Ltd, Mississauga, ON, Canada; Greek National Tourist Board, Toronto and Montreal, Canada; National Archaeological Museum, Athens, Greece; Trustees of the National Museums of Scotland, Edinburgh, Scotland; Parke-Davis, Scarborough, ON, Canada; Roman Baths Museum, Bath, England; the Content Family Collection of Ancient Cameos, Houlton, Maine, US; Grosvenor Museum, Chester, England; English Heritage; Archaeology Museum, University of Durham, England; The Royal College of Physicians and Surgeons of Canada, Ottawa, ON, Canada; The Royal Society of Medicine, London, England; Archaeologisches Institute, University of Jena, Germany; Viscount Bledisloe, Lydney Park Museum, Lydney, Gloucestershire, England; *British Journal of Ophthalmology*, London, England; The Society of Antiquaries of London, England; Tullie House City Museum and Art Gallery, Carlisle, England; The Institute of Archaeology, Oxford, England; Shrewsbury and Wroxeter Museums, Shropshire, England; Sydney Renow Esq, Esher, Surrey, England; Chesters Museum, Hadrian's Wall Museums, England; Ospedale Fatebenefratelli, Rome, Italy; Classic Numismatic Group Inc, Lancaster, PA, US and London, England; Spink and Son Ltd, London, England; and Ms Cindy Buhle, Bracebridge, ON, Canada, for preparing the drawings.

Author information

Gerald Hart graduated MD from the University of Toronto in 1952. He did six years' postgraduate training in internal medicine, haematology and oncology at the University of Toronto and the Chester Beatty Cancer Research Institute, London, England. He is a Fellow of the Royal College of Physicians of Canada and the American College of Physicians; he is also an Emeritus Member of the International Society of Hematology and a Fellow of the Royal Numismatic Society. He practised haematology and oncology at the Toronto East General Hospital where he served a period as Physician-in-Chief, and was Consultant (Haematology) to the Ontario Cancer Foundation and the Princess Margaret Hospital. He was also Associate Professor, Department of Medicine at the University of Toronto. During his career, he was President of the Academy of Medicine, Toronto, and Corresponding Vice-President of the Royal Society of Medicine. He also served as President of the Medico-Legal Society of Toronto, the Toronto Medical Historical Club and the Ancient Coin Society of Canada. He has been actively involved in writing papers related to haematology, oncology, palaeopathology, numismatics and the history of medicine. He has contributed more than 100 articles to journals and three chapters to books, and has edited a book on *Disease in Ancient Man*. He retired from medical practice in 1989 and is now settled in Dorset, England, where he continues his studies on Roman Britain, numismatics and the history of medicine. He is currently Honorary Treasurer of the Dorset Archaeology Committee.

Dr Martin Forrest has studied at the Universities of Leeds, Cambridge, Bath and Exeter. He has taught Classics and Ancient History to trainee teachers, and is currently lecturing at the University of the West of England, Bristol. He has been involved in popularizing a study of ancient Greece and Rome through the medium of English, at both school and university level, for more than 30 years.

List of illustrations

The source of the illustration is indicated in brackets; permission to reproduce the illustration has been sought where necessary — please refer to Appendix 2 for abbreviations

Preface

This book has been written to popularize Asclepius and interpret the present-day use of his staff and serpent symbol by various disciplines of the healthcare team. It offers a wide-ranging survey and discussion of the god Asclepius in the ancient world of Greece and Rome, based on first-hand evidence. The contents will be of interest to those working within or associated with the world of medicine today and to teachers and students of the history of medicine.

Asclepius, the Greek god of medicine, was not one of the 12 Great Olympians. Although he had lower status among the ancient Greek gods, he became one of the most popular deities of the ancient world — his symbol has survived into the 21st century. This book reviews Asclepian temple medicine and offers a clinical explanation for its success. Priests, not physicians, were involved with the rituals of temple medicine; however, both competent and incompetent healers were attracted to the crowds of supplicants at temple sites. This assemblage of medical practitioners would have led to discussions of medical experiences and, like today's 'medical rounds', would have improved patient care and resulted in medical progress.

Text has been drawn from literary and archaeological sources, including epigraphic and numismatic material. The inspiration for the book and much of its content stem from Dr Gerald Hart's life work as a medical practitioner and his keen interest in numismatics and the ancient world. He was encouraged to expand this unique aspect of Asclepius by Professor GR Paterson, Executive Director of the Hannah Institute for the History of Medicine and Professor Ernie Steib, Associate Dean, Faculty of Pharmacy, University of Toronto. Subject matter with clinical implications have been identified and interpreted against a background of 40 years' medical practice. The indepth involvement with classical subjects and their existing translations into noncontemporary language indicated the need for participation of an experienced classicist and teacher. Dr Martin Forrest has published extensively in these fields and has spent the past 30 years popularizing the classics. He edited the classical material and retranslated the Latin and Greek quotations.

The *Edelstein Testimonies*, published in 1945 by Emma and Ludwig Edelstein, have provided a basic, literary research source. These authors collected all known literary references and inscriptions[1] to

Asclepius, and organized them into various subject groups containing the original Greek and Latin text accompanied by a translation. They listed the original translator in their index; when no translation was available, Dr Evelyn Clift worked on this in collaboration with the authors. This new publication offers modern translations of all literary and epigraphic sources quoted while retaining the system of referencing used by the Edelsteins. In their *Testimonies*, each quote was assigned a T number, ranging from T 1 to T 861. This text will identify their reference source with ET plus the relevant number.

The Edelsteins felt the words of ancient authors reflected the overall attitude to Asclepius by the contemporary educated upper classes. Unfortunately, they considered the numerous inscriptions to him had less historical importance, and made a selection of these to prevent their work from becoming unwieldy. Their editing excluded repetitive dedications as well as reports of individual significance or only of 'local interest'; this, unfortunately, eliminated the identification of many sites of worship. However, their masterpiece of scholarly work remains a primary basic resource not only for erudite study but also for those with a general interest. I gratefully acknowledge the Johns Hopkins University Press, Baltimore, for permission to reproduce material from the *Edelstein Testimonies*.

According to Plato, the Greek philosopher, Hippocrates was the leader of the Asclepiads (followers of Asclepius). His humoral theory is reviewed which, even today, has potential for clinical application. The oath of Hippocrates is discussed in its original form as well as its usage. The old oath is devolving and some of its basic concepts are coalescing with modern ethical concepts to produce a politically correct, client-orientated mission statement with universal application for today's doctors.

In contrast to epigraphic sources, that were written for the upper classes and require the language skills of a classicist for translation and interpretation, coins were minted for everyday use by the man in the street and they afford numismatists a unique perspective for studying the gods of antiquity. Ancient coins present contemporary viewpoints of the gods and emphasize the everyday impact of religious themes. Some coins reveal the location of religious sites and even depict details of temple architecture; others portray aspects of ritual or attest to the belief in Asclepius by the current ruler. In this book, coins become an equal partner of epigraphy as a source of original information and full partner as a source of illustration. Appropriate numismatic details have been placed in the Notes and References sections so as not to interrupt the flow of text[2-4]. Due to varying photographic sources and photographs, coin sizes are not actual; the numismatic notes provide accurate details.

This review identifies 513 sites where Asclepius was worshipped. More than one-half (267) were associated with ancient coins, while numismatic evidence is the only record for 211 Asclepian temple sites.

The text also discusses the evidence of archaeological remains as well as displays and artefacts located in various museum collections. Pertinent data from major sites have also been reviewed and, where possible, reference has been made to the evidence of Asclepius in the most distant part of the Roman empire.

> 'Britain, right at the end of the earth. . . . the Britons, furthest of earth's peoples.' Horace *Odes* I, XXXV (26 BC)

The adoption of Christianity resulted in the decline and extinction of all ancient Greek and Roman religions, now regarded as pagan practices. Many of these left some imprint on Christianity, but the influence of basic medical practices and ethics associated with Asclepius survived through the era of Christian healing. During the Renaissance, these ancient theories relating to the physical factors causing sickness were rediscovered and the progress of medical science was thus reawakened. The staff of Asclepius remains the symbol of medical care today.

Throughout the book, Greek proper names and other words transliterated from the original Greek have generally been referred to in their Roman form — thus, Asclepius is used whenever Greek contexts (Asklepios) are referred to, while the Roman Aesculapius is used whenever Latin-speaking parts of the Roman empire are involved.

Notes and references

1. Edelstein EJ, Edelstein L. *Asclepius: a collection and interpretation of testimonies.* Baltimore: Johns Hopkins Press, 1945.
2. Gods and ancient coins: evolution of a practical monetary system required around 300 years. The earliest known coins were crude pellets of silver with scratch or punch marks on one side, produced in c700 BC by Lydia (part of western Turkey). Cnidus produced a silver coin with a questionable crude portrait of Apollo c700–650 BC, followed by another showing the forepart of a lion and the head of Aphrodite c650–550 BC. Royalty and aristocrats used this initial coinage as their medium for international trade but it was not accepted universally as true value. Foreign coinage was often melted so as to check its purity; this was a service for which the country of origin paid a fee (not very different from the policy of today's banks discounting the value of foreign currency transactions!). The introduction of coins for day-to-day use required a small portion of bullion of guaranteed weight and fineness that would be an acceptable replacement for bartering of goods and services. The guarantee came from the issuer's (ie state's) stamp or badge appearing on the coin, as well as a depiction of the predominant local deity. The portrait of the god located the origin of the coin and, because local kings and dynasties were often replaced by wars, rendered continuity to its value. Royal portraits did not appear on coinage until after the apotheosis of Alexander the Great as the son of Zeus in 323 BC. Coins sometimes had propaganda value—the issuing authority depicted what it wanted the man in the street to see. As early as 550 BC, King Croesus of Lydia had

portrayed on one side of a coin a bull facing a lion—a symbol of his own power. Athens was the first state to produce money for everyday use. In 560 BC, a silver coin of the state portrayed Athena on the obverse and her symbolic owl on the reverse. This coin was improved over the centuries and the Athenian silver tetradrachm (the 'Athens Owl') became the international standard for everyday currency in the ancient Mediterranean world. The gods contributed significantly to the successful introduction of a monetary system in the ancient world. Portraits of gods on coins served as a constant reminder to the ancient Greeks of a divine role in their daily lives, and study of these ancient coins attests to the reality of mythology to the people who used them. Man's universal desire to please the gods rendered coins a special place in daily living; the deities might even bless or favour transactions in which the coins were used. Fear of retribution by the gods discouraged counterfeiters. Special care was taken with the coin portraits of the gods and even today some of the finest examples of coin art are the depictions of ancient Greek gods[3]. The tradition of affording coins a religious aspect continues today with the inscription 'In God we trust' on American coins and 'DG' (by the grace of God) on British ones. When currency became firmly established, life-like portraits of rulers began to supplement or replace the gods. Mint marks and the names of moneyers were also added as a guarantee for the value of the coin. Some Roman additions to the information portrayed on coins included details about the rulers (which incidentally allow precise dating), mottoes of political value, and personifications that emphasize the virtues of the emperor and his reign. Some of these additions are described in the glossary of numismatic terms[4]. Archaeological evidence for the worship of Asclepius as depicted on coins is scattered throughout the ancient world.

3. Pictures of the best coins depicting Greek gods appear in: Kraay CM, Hirmer M, eds. *Greek coins*. London: Thames and Hudson, 1966.

4. Numismatic glossary: obverse is the principal side of the coin (heads) and reverse the opposite side (tails). Mintmark identifies the place where the coin was struck (made). Roman emperors had themselves portrayed on the obverse of their coins; both portrait and attire varied with the message they wished to convey. They squeezed into the inscription surrounding their portrait a variety of abbreviations summarizing their titles and honours: AUG (Augustus) was the most distinctive of Imperial titles. If there were two or three head rulers, the inscription would be AUGG or AUGGG respectively. Caesar or Caes was the second highest rank and denoted heir to the throne. PM, Pon M, Pon Max, Pontifex Max (Pontifex Maximus) was an emperor's title as supreme head of the Roman religion. TRP, Trib P, Trib Pot, Trib Potest (Tribunica Potestas) referred to the emperor as supreme civil head of state; it was often followed by a number that signified the years served in this office (this is one of the most useful keys to date a coin). COS is a short form for consul, one of the two chief magistrates of the Roman state; it was also often followed by a number. PP (PATER PATRIAE) meant father of the country; IMP (IMPERATOR) meant emperor. The first and middle names were usually abbreviated. From this information, it is possible to date the year of minting (actual dates did not appear on coins until the 15th century). The reverse of Roman coins portrayed a deity, a personification or a symbol. Frequently, these had some type of propaganda value; for instance, Concordia seems to appear after a period of internal strife and Fel Temp Rep, the ancient equivalent of 'happy times are here again', was an effort to reassure the public that the government had matters in hand. Greek coins had an additional mini-design peripheral to the main symbol, indicating the magistrate responsible for minting the coin. For those interested in further reading, many numismatic publications exist that cover all aspects of coinage and are suitable for both beginners and experts. Some coin illustrations in this text are accompanied by numismatic details: AU, AR, AE are abbreviations for gold, silver and bronze respectively; the number that follows indicates either the diameter of the coin or its weight.

Chapter 1

Asclepius — from myth to reality

Birth of mythology

Communities inhabiting the earth in antiquity believed that supernatural forces controlled their daily lives. They humanized these invisible powers into divine and semi-human beings — their concepts became the communities' gods who inhabited the sky, earth, waters and underworld. They attributed storms, pestilence and disasters to the displeasure of gods and, conversely, credited fulfilment of their daily needs and success of their endeavours as a sign of favour from the gods. It was generally accepted that these invisible beings had to be propitiated with gestures of thanks in the form of gifts and sacrifices on every possible occasion. Rituals were performed at locally assigned, terrestrial homes for their gods — these were located on lofty hilltops, in groves, at wells, springs and rivers, and in caves, fissures and deep shafts[1,2]. These ancient and diverse holy places acquired an aura of sanctity that remains to the present day. Stories concerning the creation of the gods were evolved and these legends became the basis of folk mythology. Myths also developed, which were used to explain natural phenomena such as day and night, the seasons, weather changes, and natural catastrophes such as earthquakes and violent storms.

Greek and Roman mythology

When the early Greek and Latin peoples migrated southwards in about 2000 BC, they brought with them their shared Indo-European beliefs about their gods. Once established in the mainland of Greece and the Italian peninsula respectively, the Greeks and Romans shared many similar mythological concepts. However, they did not speak a common language which led to their mutual deities acquiring different names. For instance, the goddess of grain and harvest was called Demeter by the Greeks and Ceres by the Romans, while Zeus was Greek king of the gods who was known as Jupiter in the Roman world. One exception was the god Apollo, whose name was common to both peoples.

Greeks and Romans both believed their gods possessed human form but were of larger stature. The gods enjoyed, or were susceptible to, many human frailties, especially sins of the flesh. They maintained a

1

personal interest in the welfare of mortal men and women, but were stern and would punish humans for disbelief, greed, arrogance and ingratitude. It was thought that the gods lived at the top of Mount Olympus, whose peak in north eastern Greece even today often assumes mysterious distortions due to mist and mirage. The mountain's height of more than 2,900 metres is enhanced visually by the disposition of the sea and surrounding hills. This monument of nature was considered to be the throne of Zeus and 'heavenly' home of the major Greek gods.

There were said to be 12 main Olympian deities in the Greek and Roman pantheon, each playing a major role in human affairs[3,4,5] (Table 1). Many other deities presided over different aspects of life and could be linked to the Olympian gods. Among them was Asclepius (Aesculapius to the Romans), thought to be the son of Olympian Apollo. Apollo was often referred to as Phoebus Apollo and was regarded as god of healing, prophecy, poetry and music. Despite associating their gods with the upper reaches of Mount Olympus, the ancient Greeks also referred to other gods as 'chthonian' (gods of the earth) who were associated with the underworld. Hades, the underworld equivalent to Olympian Zeus, ruled the underworld where the souls of mortals went after death. Persephone was the daughter of Demeter, the Olympian goddess of grain and harvest, who was abducted by and compelled to live with Hades for six months.

There were also many lesser deities, such as nymphs, who were generally associated with specific locations on the earth and 'hero-gods'. Heracles (the Roman Hercules) is one of the best remembered hero-gods. He had once been a mortal ruler famed for his heroic exploits and was worshipped as a god by the Greeks and Romans. Myths describing the origins of the gods had regional variations based on local legends. The Greeks and Romans tolerated these inconsistencies and, with the expansion of trade and colonization, often encountered new, local deities who were frequently adopted into their own family of gods. The expanding scope of human endeavour created the need for new gods dedicated to these areas of human need. Expanding Greek civilization required a god of medicine who would be dedicated to the bringing of good health and the relief of suffering.

Asclepius the physician
Asclepius was the Greek god of healing and medicine. Literary evidence indicates that Asclepius was a real person whose deeds

enabled him to become a hero-god. The increasing need for a god dedicated to the ills of mankind resulted in the evolution of an Olympian god of medicine.

The earliest record of his name appears in Homer's *Iliad*, whose central story is located in the siege of Troy by the Achaeans (Greeks). Its text is believed to have broadly existed in its present form in the latter half of the eighth century BC. Wace and Stubbings suggest that the catalogue of ships in Book II of the *Iliad* portrays the 'Achaean' world of early Greece, as well as its constituent states, rulers and the relative size of its communities[6]. In this setting, Asclepius and his two physician sons, Machaon and Podalirius, appear to be real human beings, closely associated with Tricca in the north eastern Greek region of Thessaly:

'And those who lived in Tricca and craggy Ithome and those who lived in Oechalia, city of Oechalian Eurytus, these again were led by the two sons of Asclepius, the skilled doctors, Podalirius and Machaon. And with these were lined up thirty hollow ships'. (Homer, *Iliad* 729–32)[7]

It has been argued that Asclepius, as referred to in the Homeric poems, is undoubtedly a renowned healer who passed his skill on to his sons. Archaeological evidence supports Homer's tale of Troy. In the 1870s and 1880s, the German entrepreneur and amateur archaeologist, Heinrich Schliemann, searched for Homer's city and excavated the mound of Hisarlik in Turkey — the suspected site of ancient Troy. Schliemann revealed that this was the site of a city of great antiquity, which flourished in the third and second millennia BC. He claimed he had found living proof of many features of the city described in the *Iliad*. Subsequent excavations by Dorpfeld in the 1890s, Blegen of the University of Cincinatti (1932–8) and, very recently, by an international team led by Korfmann have added to and modified Schliemann's original findings[8,9]. Excavations have revealed more than 46 building phases, including the walled citadel known as Troy VI and its successor, Troy VIIa. Both cities came to a violent end — Troy VIIa shows evidence of preparations for a siege — and were contemporary with the last years of Mycenaean (early Greek) civilization that flourished in mainland Greece during the late Bronze Age. Recent study has shown further evidence for Mycenaean contacts with Troy. If we are seeking evidence for the Trojan War as an historical event, this is its likely historical context, with Homer's 'Achaeans' identified with the Mycenaean Greeks.

Although many scholars would urge caution, it is generally accepted that the Greek legends of a Trojan War contain some residue of reality. This poses the question of whether or not it is possible, or likely, that some of the participants in Homer's *Iliad* were real historical figures. In the Trojan War, Asclepius is referred to as 'the blameless physician' whose sons, Machaon and Podalirius, led the contingent from Tricca in the *Iliad's* catalogue of Greek ships. If Asclepius had performed deeds of heroic proportions, then he could have been deified as a hero-god, thereby supporting chronologically the claim that Hippocrates was his 18th descendant (ET 215).

Asclepius the hero-god
In addition to mythological gods, the ancient Greeks believed in apotheosized mortals whom they regarded as hero-gods[10]. Although deceased, they were worshipped as powerful individuals and were thought to exist in a halfway state between gods and ordinary mortal beings. The hero-gods had been founders of cities and colonies, famous rulers and military leaders, and had often performed great super-human feats. The best known among them is Heracles. Much evidence suggests that Asclepius should be included in this category.

Hero-gods beneficially influenced mortal affairs but had to be recognized, worshipped and given sacrifices. Ritual observances were probably of an ancient chthonian origin and contrasted with worship of the Olympian gods, to whom pure white, sacrificial victims were offered during daylight hours. Chthonian deity worship involved sacrifices made during the hours of darkness. Dark-skinned animals were burnt and sacrificed over low altars, and their blood was allowed to drain into the soil.

In the *Iliad*, Asclepius is described as the earthly ruler of the community of Tricca — he is also referred to as a physician whose two sons led a contingent of men and ships in the Trojan expedition. Asclepius might have been the first human physician to be deified which, if correct, may explain his association with the Egyptian, Imhotep. As physician, architect and vizier to the Egyptian Pharaoh Netjerket (Djoser) of the third dynasty (c2686–13 BC), Imhotep experienced apotheosis possibly as early as the 19th dynasty (c1295–1186 BC) but certainly by the 27th dynasty (525–404 BC), and became the Egyptian god of medicine. When Egypt was ruled by the Ptolemies, the Greeks who had settled in Egypt called him Imouthis and identified him with Asclepius; his tomb at Memphis became one of the most famous of Asclepian centres[11].

Celsus supported the hero-god status for Asclepius when, in the first century AD, he wrote in the introduction to his *De Medicina*: 'Hence Aesculapius, though he is recognised as its most ancient founder and because he brought to this science [of medicine], which was still crude and in its infancy, a greater degree of precision, was given a place among the gods'. (ET 244)

The etymology of Asclepius has been credited to several earthly origins suggesting the existence of a real physician by that name:

'The name Asclepius derives from "to heal gently" and from "deferring the withering that comes with death".' (ET 268)[12]

'... the name Asclepius comes from this word [dried up] ... together with the word for gentleness, that is, he who with the aid of his medical skills does not allow dryness.' (ET 269)

Withering and dryness refer to dehydration, a frequent cause of death before intravenous therapy was possible. Other sources refer to a specific event:

'... Asclepius was originally called Epios, because of his gentleness and calmness, but was named Asclepius after he had cured Ascles, the tyrant of Epidaurus, of ophthalmia.' (ET 271)

Another reference to this last episode calls Asclepius 'The one who soothed the dryness associated with illnesses'. (ET 273)

Emma and Ludwig Edelstein, authors of the *Edelstein Testimonies*[13] which provides references and inscriptions to Asclepius, concluded that Asclepius was a demi-god or hero-god created by men in order to have someone in charge of healing. Galen, the famous second century physician to the Roman Emperor Marcus Aurelius, appears to be ambivalent in his statements. In a plea to the deity to heal the emperor, he appears to describe Asclepius as a 'demi-god', using the word 'daemon' rather than 'theos', the word for god[13]:

'Have mercy, Blessed healer, you who created this remedy, whether you inhabit the hilly ridges of Tricca, O demi-god, or in Rhodes or in Cos or in Epidaurus by the sea. Have mercy and send your ever kindly daughter, Panacea, to the Emperor, who will offer you sacrifices of good omen for ridding him once and for all from his pain.' (*De Antidotis*, I, 6 XIV, p 42 K) (ET 595)

However, Galen elsewhere acknowledges Asclepius as a full-blown mythological god and distinguishes him from mortal heroes (*Introduction*, Cp 1 XIX, p674K) (ET 356):

'The Greeks ascribe the creation of the arts either to the children of the gods or to certain men akin to them to whom the gods first imparted every art. So they say that the art of medicine was first learned by Asclepius from Apollo, his father, and then transmitted to mankind; for this reason he is considered to be the discoverer of it. Before Asclepius, the medical art did not yet exist among men, but men of old had some experience with drugs and herbs, such as those that, among the Greeks, Chiron the Centaur and the heroes, who were instructed by him, knew well....'

The debate about the historicity of the Trojan War continues to this date[14]. However, if we refer to evidence in Homer's *Iliad*, dating from the late eighth century BC and, in particular, to his description of the treatment of the wounded Menelaus by one of Asclepius' sons, it would appear that, at the time, Asclepius was regarded as a great earthly physician who had acquired his knowledge of drugs from Chiron. This statement places the origin of Asclepius the demi-god in the second half of the eighth century BC. The existing text of the *Iliad*, however, is known to contain fossilized memories of earlier times and recollections of a mortal healer called Asclepius may go back even further than this.

Graf suggests that, as a hero-god, Asclepius was more easily accessible than Apollo who could 'proclaim lofty indifference towards man and his destiny'; even as a god, he suggests, Asclepius was never so distant. Another modern historian, Papadakis, believes that Asclepius was a hero who reached divine status over time. He participated in both the human and the divine natures and the god and hero-god Asclepius were worshipped separately. He suggests that the tholos of Epidaurus was the burial place of the hero-god Asclepius and a shrine where he was worshipped[15].

A current analogy of the hero-god concept occurs with Christianity's description of Jesus as man and god.

Asclepius the Olympian god

We hear of Asclepius as a legendary figure in the Greek lyric poetry of Pindar but, by the mid-fifth century BC, an elaborate mythology had been built up around the origin of Asclepius. In Pindar's version of the story (*Pythiae* II, 1–58; ET 1), Asclepius was the son of the god Phoebus Apollo and of the mortal princess Coronis, daughter of Phlegyas who was the ruler of Thessaly. Much later, the Roman poet Ovid (43 BC–17 AD), followed the tradition that Asclepius came from northern Greece and included a detailed account of the Asclepius story in his *Metamorphoses*. This entire work was a catalogue of the Graeco-Roman legends and myths involving miraculous transformations, from the creation of the world onwards. Ovid's version of the Asclepius story will be used here as the basic text for this myth (ET 2).

Both Pindar and Ovid describe the story of how the baby Asclepius was removed from his mother's womb as her corpse was about to be consumed in flames.

'In the whole of Thessaly, no one was more beautiful than Coronis of Larissa. It is a fact that the god of Delphi, Apollo, was in love with her, as long as there was no one else in her love life, or at least, as long as she was able to deceive him! But Apollo's bird, the raven, discovered her unfaithfulness and the single-minded tell-tale rushed off to tell his master about the wrong-doing that he had discovered... The bird continued on his way and told Apollo that he had seen Coronis in bed with a young man from Thessaly. The moment that he heard this accusation, Apollo's laurel wreath slipped from his head, the colour drained from his cheeks and his plectrum fell from his hand. His mind welled up with anger. He reached for his usual weapons: he strung his bow, bending it from the horns, and shot an unerring arrow straight through the very breast that had so often been pressed against his own. Coronis cried out in agony as the arrow struck home; she drew it out and as she did so, bright red blood spurted out all over her white limbs. "Phoebus Apollo", she cried, "I have deserved this punishment, but why could you not let me first give birth to our child? Now the two of us [the child and I] will die together." Those were her last words and with that, her life ebbed away as her blood oozed out. A deathly cold spread over her lifeless body. Then her lover was filled with remorse for the cruel punishment he had exacted on her, but it was too late. He was filled with hatred against himself for listening to the tale and for allowing himself to flare up with anger in the way he had done. He hated the bird that had told him of Coronis' guilt and had thus caused him to be so upset. He hated the bow and his hand and the arrows that his hands had so rashly unleashed. He massaged her lifeless body in an attempt to keep the Fates at bay, but his assistance came too late. He used his skills as a healer to no avail. When he realised that his efforts

were in vain, that the funeral pyre was all ready and that her limbs
were about to be consumed in flames, Apollo groaned from the very
depths of his heart, for the gods are forbidden to moisten their
cheeks with tears. He sounded just like a young cow who sees the
hammer poised close to the right ear of the slaughterman come
crashing down with a mighty blow upon the hollow forehead of an
unweaned calf. The God then poured perfumes which she would
never be able to enjoy, over Coronis' breast. He embraced her for
the last time and then performed the funeral ceremonies that were
for her so untimely. To prevent his own offspring from disappearing
among the ashes, he snatched his child from his mother's womb and
from the flames and took him away to the cave of the centaur
Chiron. As for the raven, he was expecting to be rewarded for letting
Apollo know the truth. Instead, the God forbade him from ever
being a bird of white plumage again. Meanwhile, the centaur was
thrilled to have the son of a god to look after; he felt honoured to be
given this task. Suddenly, his daughter arrived, her reddish gold hair
streaming over her shoulders. This daughter was his child by the
nymph Cariclo, who had called her Ocyrhoe, after the rushing
stream on whose banks she had been born. Not content merely to
learn her father's arts, she was able to foretell the future. So when
she felt a prophetic frenzy seizing hold of her mind and had grown
warm with the divine presence that burned within her, she looked on
the baby and cried: "Little boy, bringer of health to the whole world,
may you grow up and flourish! Mortals will often owe their lives to
you and you will be given the right to bring back to life those that
have already died. But one day, you will make the gods angry by
your daring and will be prevented by your grandfather's thunderbolt
from ever doing such a thing again. From being an immortal god,
you will be reduced to a lifeless corpse, but later, from this corpse,
you will once again become a god and, for the second time, you will
renew your destiny." ' (ET 2)

The role of the raven is confirmed by Hesiod (ET 22) and his fate
confirmed by Apollodorus, writing in the third century BC (ET 3):
'Apollo cursed the raven that brought the news and turned him black
instead of the white colour he had been before'.
The mythographer, Apollodorus, also provides further detail
concerning Asclepius:

'Having become a surgeon and having developed his skills to a high
degree, he not only prevented some people from dying, but even

brought them back to life. For he had received from Athena the blood that had flowed from the veins of the Gorgon, and while he could use the blood that flowed from her left side to take away human life, he used the blood from her right side to bring them back to life. This is how he managed to raise people from the dead.... But Zeus, fearing that people might learn this healing art from him, and so rescue one another from death, struck Asclepius with a thunderbolt. In order to get his own back, Apollo slew the Cyclopes, who had manufactured the thunderbolt for Zeus.'

Diodorus, writing in the late first century BC, expanded further the reasons for the anger of Zeus:

'Asclepius' reputation became so great that he cured many who had not expected to recover and this is why he seemed to have brought so many back to life. This is the origin of the story that even Hades brought a charge against Asclepius, accusing him before Zeus on the grounds that he was losing his powers; for the dead were constantly becoming fewer, because they were being healed by Asclepius.' (ET 4)

With the exception of Homer, these writers from classical antiquity tell us that Asclepius was the son of Apollo. His beautiful mortal mother, Coronis, lived in Thessaly; in a fit of rage, Apollo changed the colour of the raven's plumage from white to black because it had been the messenger of Coronis' infidelity. Apollo was unable to resuscitate Coronis who had died bleeding profusely from an arrow wound in the chest—a case of exsanguination. Today, even with modern treatment methods and transfusion, similar wounds are frequently fatal. Asclepius was delivered by Caesarean section and was adopted by Chiron, the centaur, whose daughter, Ocyrhoe, prophesied that Asclepius would become a skilled physician who would bring the dead back to life but would be punished by Zeus. He, too, would be resurrected and was destined to continue pursuing his medical practice[16].

Chiron was said to act as official foster parent on behalf of the gods. Other sources indicate that Chiron was highly educated in every branch of knowledge. He is famed for having educated some of the famous heroes of ancient Greece, including: Jason who sailed in search of the golden fleece; Achilles, the central heroic figure in the *Iliad*; Achilles' father, Peleus; Heracles; and Asclepius. He is credited with teaching Achilles to play the lyre, Heracles astronomy and Asclepius medicine.

Asclepius was the first to institute the practice of surgery and the art of pharmacology (ET 61). Other sources reveal that he acquired these by using herbs that had been spilt on the Thessalian Plain by the sorceress, Medea (ET 282, 15) (Hyginus, *Fabulae*, CCLXIV 9, ET 360). Chiron taught Asclepius all his medical skills; while under Chiron's tutelage, he tended the serpents on Mount Pelion, who taught him their secret knowledge of herbs.

Asclepius attracted the favour of Athena, who gave him some of the Gorgon's blood which possessed the power to revive the dead[17]. Asclepius' treatment successes with this gift angered Hades, who complained to Zeus that his realm was in danger of being starved of newly recruited dead. Zeus found the complaint to be valid and his judgement was harsh. Asclepius was first suspended from medical practice and then punished by death from a thunderbolt. Apollo objected to Zeus' action but, because there was no right of appeal, he took the law into his own hands and retaliated by killing the Cyclopes, the three one-eyed giants, who had forged Zeus' special thunderbolts. Zeus subsequently mollified Apollo's anger by granting Asclepius the honour of becoming a new constellation within the constellation of Scorpion (ET 121). Unfortunately, no mythological or other source records Asclepius' return to medical practice on earth. Presumably, Apollo's violent protests influenced Zeus to resurrect Asclepius, who returned to earth in the role of god of medicine, but was restrained by a caveat which prohibited him from reviving the dead[18].

The myth of Asclepius had several local versions and his birthplace was claimed by a number of communities. These included Tricca in Thessaly, previously mentioned (ET 11), Messenia (ET 16), Arcadia (ET 17) and Epidaurus which made the most successful claim by using the ancient Bronze Age hill sanctuary of Apollo Maleatas, god of healing. The Epidaurians believed that Asclepius had been suckled by a goat and guarded by the herd's watchdog on the slopes of a mountain known as Mount Nipple (ET 7). The Museum of Epidaurus today holds a third century BC stele bearing an inscription to Apollo and Asclepius, erected by Isyllos to commemorate the origin in the temple (*hieron*) of Epidaurus.

There are other versions of the birth of Asclepius. Hesiod, writing in around 700 BC, refers to Asclepius' mother as Arsinoe from Messenia in southern Greece. Some sources state that Hermes performed the Caesarean section, and Pindar credited Artemis with the slaying of Coronis (ET 1). The Christian Bishop Theodoret, in his early fifth century AD summary of the myth, implied that Asclepius had a spontaneous delivery. He was then secretly abandoned by Coronis on

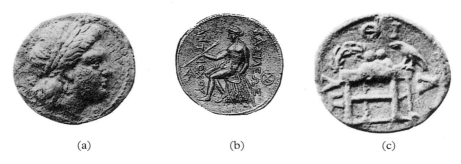

(a) (b) (c)

Figure 1
(a) Apollo depicted on the obverse of a coin from Epidaurus (fourth century BC); the reverse of this coin depicts the Thrasymedes statue of Asclepius shown in Figure 6 (BMC, M&W)
(b) A coin from Syria (270–267 BC) which depicts a nude and somewhat effeminate Apollo seated on an omphalos. His right hand holds one of his lethal arrows, his left hand the top of his bow (CNG)
(c) A bronze coin of Epidaurus (146–75 AD) which depicts the raven symbolic of Apollo with the inscription Pythia (the priestess who officiated at the prophetic cave of Delphi) (BMC, M&W)

the mountainside near Epidaurus, where he was nurtured by a dog and later found by hunters who took him to Chiron (ET 5). Another version located his birthplace in the sacred grove of Epidaurus with Artemis and the Fates (who were said to spin the thread of life and eventually cut it off) attending his birth as midwives.

Reality of the Asclepian myth
People of ancient Greece and Rome recognized the gods from their portraits on everyday coinage, and by their depiction in paintings, statues and pottery. The gods involved in the Asclepian myth were familiar to all.

There were many depictions of Apollo, often symbolized by a bow and arrow — his punishment of the raven was remembered on a coin of Epidaurus (Figure 1). Even today, visitors to his famous sanctuary at Delphi are reminded of his rage and punishment of the raven. Admission tickets to Delphi depict a white drinking cup from 470 BC portraying Apollo seated facing a black raven (Figure 2). Coins throughout antiquity, originating from different places in the ancient world, portrayed the other participants in the Asclepian Myth and enhanced the reality of his presence in everyday life. Coronis appeared on a coin minted in the name of Sabina, the childless wife of the Emperor Hadrian[19]; other gods in the myth (Hades, Zeus, Athena) as

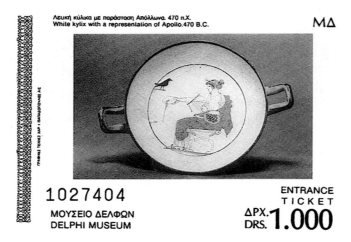

Λευκή κύλικα με παράσταση Απόλλωνα. 470 π.Χ.
White kylix with a representation of Apollo.470 B.C.

ΜΔ

1027404

ΜΟΥΣΕΙΟ ΔΕΛΦΩΝ
DELPHI MUSEUM

ENTRANCE
TICKET

ΔΡΧ.
DRS.1.000

Figure 2 Modern ticket of admission to the temple of Apollo at Delphi. The kylix (drinking cup) shows Apollo seated facing a black raven

well as Chiron and the monstrous Gorgon were also familiar coin portraits (Figure 3).

Asclepius is portrayed on many coins from the fifth century BC to the fourth century AD. His likeness on coins augmented the reality of his presence to those using the money and served as a handy talisman for prayer. Asclepius was shown with a mature face, a beard and a full head of curly hair (Figure 4). Although his portrait resembles that of Zeus, Asclepius had a demeanour more kindly than stern; there was often a smooth or twisted headband below his hair. In contrast to the nudity of the Olympian gods, he wore a regular male garment known as a *himation*. He wore this draped over his left shoulder with his right chest exposed (Figure 5). His sartorial standard is supported in Hippocrates' advice that physicians must be clean and well dressed. The most famous statue of Asclepius, executed in marble, gold and ivory, was made by Thrasymedes for the Asclepian sanctuary at Epidaurus; it depicted Asclepius seated with a dog under his throne and a serpent rising at his right side. This artistic masterpiece of the ancient world has been lost but its form, like photographs of buildings destroyed in World War Two, has been preserved on a coin from Epidaurus c350 BC (Figure 6a).

Larissa in Thessaly has a close geographical association with Tricca and was the first city in the ancient world to depict Asclepius on its coins (450–400 BC) (Figure 6b). Coins depicting Asclepius continued to circulate throughout the ancient world for more than 700 years. The

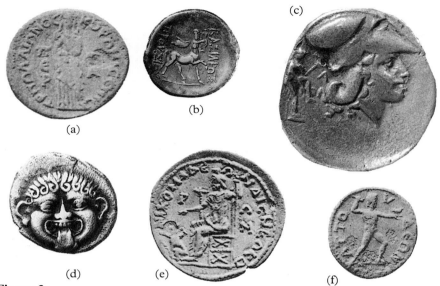

Figure 3

(a) Coronis minted by Hadrian in the name of his wife Sabina from Pergamum (117–37 AD) (GDH)

(b) Chiron holding a lyre from Bithynia (117–37 AD) (GDH)

(c) Athena as depicted on coins of Corinth and the Corinthian Colonies (350–300 BC) (GDH)

(d) Gorgon depicted on the obverse of an AR Hemidrachm from Neapolis in Macedonia (around fifth to fourth century BC) (CNG)

(e) Hades (BMC, M&W)

(f) Zeus hurling a thunderbolt from Attuda in Caria (193–211 AD) (BMC, M&W)

ready availability of these coins today indicates that large numbers must have been struck in ancient times. Such coins provided a constant reminder to contemporary populations of the healing powers of Asclepius and attested to his reality in their daily lives.

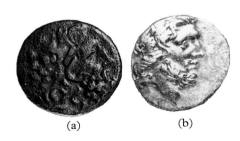

Figure 4

(a) Mature face of Asclepius from Pergamum (133 BC–Augustus) (GDH)

(b) Mature face of Asclepius from Cos (166–88 BC) (GDH)

Philippus Senior I (244–9 AD) minted a coin at Bizra which depicts the official Asclepian myth. This coin portrays Apollo in the centre with Asclepius on his right and his daughter, Hygieia, on his left; above is Zeus hurling a thunderbolt. The depiction of Fortuna, to the right of Zeus, had double symbolism; medical

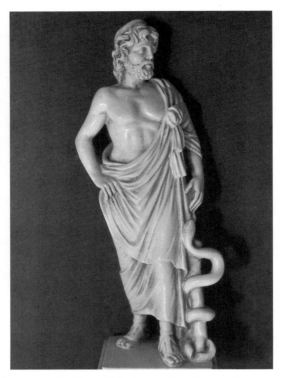

Figure 5   Modern reproduction of Asclepius based on a Roman reproduction of a classical Greek statue (21 cm high) (GDH)

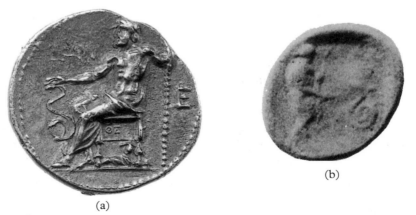

(a)   (b)

Figure 6
(a) Thrasymedes' famous chryselephantine statue of Asclepius at Epidaurus (Peloponnesus), showing Asclepius seated on a throne with a sceptre in his left hand; his right hand rests on the head of his serpent; and a dog lies beside him (323–240 BC). (Photo © Bibliothèque Nationale de France, Service Photographique, Paris, France)
(b) Asclepius feeding his serpent depicted by a coin from Larissa 450–400 BC. This is the earliest known numismatic depiction of Asclepius and adds probable significance to the fact that Hippocrates wished to be buried at Larissa (BMC, M&W)

(a)

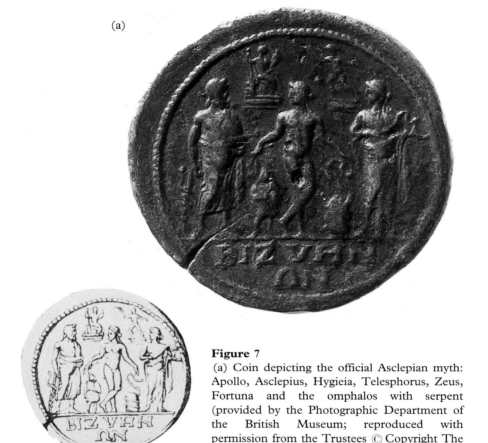

(b)

Figure 7
(a) Coin depicting the official Asclepian myth: Apollo, Asclepius, Hygieia, Telesphorus, Zeus, Fortuna and the omphalos with serpent (provided by the Photographic Department of the British Museum; reproduced with permission from the Trustees © Copyright The British Museum)
(b) A line drawing of details of 7a (BMC, M&W)

practice, past and present, requires a degree of good luck but, in addition, Fortuna protected naked bodies (a reference also to physical examination). Telesphorus, Asclepius' son and a later addition to the myth (c100 AD), is depicted with an omphalos on his left, to the right of Apollo. This coin is one of many fine third century AD depictions of Asclepius. Apollo was given precedence in the portraiture, just like formal family pictures today, in which the most senior members of the family are given greater prominence. Above the family group is Zeus hurling a thunderbolt, a grim reminder of the myth. This coin records the official Roman view of Aesculapius in the third century (Figure 7).

Other coins depicting Asclepius in the presence of fellow gods suggest his true divine status. He has been paired with Jupiter, Apollo,

Table 1   The 12 Olympians

Greek name	Roman name	Human endeavour	Medical role
Zeus	Jupiter	Sky	none assigned
Hera	Juno	Marriage	Childbirth
Poseidon	Neptune	Sea	none assigned
Demeter	Ceres	Corn, harvest	Nutrition
Apollo	Apollo	Music, hunt, prophesy	Eye, plague
Artemis	Diana	Hunting, virginity	Pregnancy
Hermes	Mercury	Commerce, messenger	Epidemics, leg
Athena	Minerva	Wisdom, art, craft and skills of the instrument maker	Healing (bath) ? = Hygieia
Hephaestus	Vulcan	The blacksmith	none assigned
Aphrodite	Venus	Love	Libido
Ares	Mars	War	none assigned
Dionysus	Liber (Bacchus)	Wine	Tonic, analgesia
Other deities:			
Hades (Pluto)	Dis	Underworld	Death
Eros	Cupido	Love	
Helius	Sol	Sun	Hot springs
Selene	Luna	Moon	
Persephone	Proserpina	Springtime	
Asclepius	Aesculapius	Medicine	Saviour
Hygieia	Salus	Health	Minerva medica, Valetudo
Hestia	Vesta	The hearth	Heat and warmth in the home

Artemis, Demeter and even had the good fortune to appear beside Aphrodite of Cnidus[20]. Other divine companions include Serapis, Nemesis and Nice. No other hero-gods were depicted on coins alongside so many Olympian companions. Ovid gave strong voice to the origin of Asclepius when he described in *Fasti*, I, 290–4, the dedication of the temple of Jupiter and Asclepius in Rome: 'The temples of the mighty grandfather and grandson are joined together'. (ET 855)

Summary

Homer's epic poem, the *Iliad*, described Asclepius as a physician whose sons were at the siege of Troy. Archaeologists have confirmed the location of Troy and found evidence of a siege having taken place. There is also evidence for Asclepius being a physician at a date no later than the eighth century BC. Asclepius' achievements led to his elevation to divine status and becoming a hero- or demi-god. After the sixth century BC, healthcare demands in ancient Greek society created the need for a god of Olympian stature and an appropriate myth evolved identifying Asclepius as an Olympian god of medicine. Ancient coins and archaeological remains emphasize the mythological origin of Asclepius and attest to his reality in the everyday lives of ordinary Greeks and Romans.

Notes and references

1. Davies H. *A walk along the wall*. London: Weidenfeld and Nicolson, 1974.
2. Cunliffe B. *The Celtic world*. New York: McGraw-Hill Publishing, 1979.
3. Seltman C. *The twelve Olympians*. Pan Books, 1961.
4. Guirand F. *Encyclopaedia of mythology*. London: Batsworth Press Ltd, 1959.
5. Webster G. *The British Celts and their gods under Rome*. London: BT Batsford Ltd, 1986.
6. Wace AJB, Stubbings FH. *Companion to Homer*. Macmillan: 1962: 52.
7. ET 10 comprises lines 729–31.
8. Blegen CW. *Troy and the Trojans*. Thames and Hudson: 1963.
9. Korfmann M *et al*. *Studia Troica*, Vols I–IV (1991/2/3/4), Verlag, Philip von Zabern, Mainz am Rhein.
10. *Encyclopaedia Britannica*. 1946; **11**: 508.
11. Emery WB. *The search for Imhotep*. London: News, Arch Section no 22157, 1965.
12. Spencer WG. *Celsus, de Medicina*. Massachusetts 1960: vol 14.
13. Edelstein EJ, Edelstein L. *Asclepius: a collection and interpretation of testimonies*. Baltimore: Johns Hopkins Press, 1945. The Edelsteins translated the word 'daemon' used here by Galen as 'demi-god'. Certainly, when the words 'theos' and daemon are used together, the latter term implies gods or lesser status or demi-gods.
14. Finley MI. Lost: the Trojan war. In: *Aspects of antiquity*. London: Chatto & Windus, 1968.
15. Papadakis T. *Epidauros: the sanctuary of Asclepius*. 7th edn. Zurich: Verlag, Schnell and Steiner, 1988.
16. This is the earliest reference to birth by Caesarean section. In ancient times, people delivered in this way were credited with divine or royal origins. The Roman historian, Pliny the Elder, falsely assigned this type of birth to Scipio and Julius Caesar. This led to the misconception that Caesarean section derived from Julius Caesar. The correct derivation comes from the Latin verb 'caedere' meaning to cut, and describes the method of delivery. This subject was reviewed by: Haggard HW. *Devils, drugs and doctors*. New York: Blue Ribbon Books, 1929. Haggard stated that 'the name Caesarian attached to it [the operation] has given rise to the belief that Julius Caesar was brought into the world by this means, but at the time when Caesar lived the operation is not known to have been performed on a living woman. His mother, Julia, lived many years after his birth, as is proven by his letters to her. The probable explanation for the name is as follows. In 715 BC the king, Numa Pompilius, codified the Roman law, and in the lex regia, as it was called, it was ordered that the child should be removed from every woman who died in far advanced pregnancy, even in cases where there was no chance of survival for the child, so that the mother and child might be buried separately. The lex regia became the lex Cesare under the rule of the emperors, and the operation became known as the caesarian operation, or section. Few such operations had been performed on living women at the time of Ambroise Paré, the father of

modern surgery (1517?–90); and for centuries after, the suffering it entailed and high mortality that resulted from it made the operation one of last resort'.

17. Gorgon blood from the right side had power to revive the dead but blood from the left side was the bane of mankind. Blood transfusions continue to be a mixed blessing. Donor blood infected by the hepatitis or AIDs virus may cause serious disease or death and becomes the modern 'bane of mankind'.

18. Routine quality control of hospital medical care includes a regular review of deaths. This process involves studying the records of deceased patients. Reviewers compare clinical diagnosis with pathological findings. They discuss the treatment and clinical course to learn more about disease, broaden clinical experience and improve patient care. The ancient literature on Asclepius allowed a medical audit of his restorations to life. Apollodorus in *Bibliotheca* III, 10, (ET 70) carried out a literature review and found the following references listed by author, (*journal*) and patient name: Stesichorus (*Eriphyle*) Capaneus and Lycurgus; (*Naupactica*) Hippolytus; Panyassis Tyndareus; Orphics, Hymenaeus; Amelesagoras, Glaucus, son of Minos. Pausanias, the Roman travel historian, recorded in *Descriptio Graecae* II, 27 (ET 739) one such case from Epidaurus in the second century AD: Apart from the others stands an ancient tablet; it says that Hippolytus dedicated 20 horses to the god. The people of Aricia have a verbal record agreeing with the inscription on this tablet. When Hippolytus was done to death by the curses of Theseus, Asclepius raised him from the dead; on coming to life again, Hippolytus refused to forgive his father and, disregarding his entreaties, went away to Aricia, Italy. There he reigned, and consecrated to Artemis a precinct, where down to my time there were contests in single combat and the victor became a priest of the goddess. The competition was not open to free men, but only to slaves who had run away from their masters. (The details of the death of Hippolytus appear in the play by the same name written by Euripides and first performed in 428 BC.)

19. The portrayal of Asclepius' mother might have been an attempt by Sabina, the childless wife of Emperor Hadrian, to propitiate Asclepius in order to conceive an heir to the throne.

20. The statue of Aphrodite at Cnidus, executed by Praxiteles, was one of the masterpieces of classical Greek art. The coin was copied from it.

---- Chapter 2 ----

The divine doctors

Apollo was foremost among the many Graeco-Roman gods who had medical skills and was the original god associated with human healthcare[1]. He was the patron god of many human endeavours but, due to the expansion of civilization, a god dedicated solely to medical care was needed. The Greeks were familiar with Asclepius, the hero-god and physician of the *Iliad*, and selected him for this role. The magnitude of this role required Olympian credentials and an appropriate Asclepian myth was created. The task was too great for Asclepius alone and so help of his family was enlisted. His family — wife, sons and daughters — all became members of the healthcare team. The divine family also expanded metaphorically when every physician adopted the title Asclepiad — son of Asclepius.

Some other Olympians maintained their specialized healing roles, in particular Athena (Minerva) and Hermes (Mercury). The Greeks eventually acquired a divine healthcare team led by Asclepius, but were still able to choose from the services of other gods.

Apollo Medicus
The Greeks and Romans recognized Apollo from his many depictions on statues and coins — these displayed his nudity and emphasized an athletic physique with the idealized beauty of youth. His face was beardless, forehead high and his long hair sometimes fell over his back or was knotted on top or at the nape of the neck with two locks tumbling over his shoulders (Figures 1b & 8).

A few of Apollo's many services to mankind were selected at some places of worship — these were often indicated by including a specific attribute to his local statues and coins. God of the hunt and hounds was one of his predominant early roles. This activity was shown on statues by a bow and arrow, and on local coins by portraying a facial image on the obverse and a bow and quiver or arrows on the reverse. In this role, he acquired the epithet 'Apollo Maleatas' (Figures 1b & 9a). His role as god of music was indicated by statues portraying him with a lyre, an instrument also shown on the reverse of his coins. Similarly, a shepherd's crook indicated his role as god of flocks and shepherds. His favourite, and most remunerative, role was as god of prophecy and

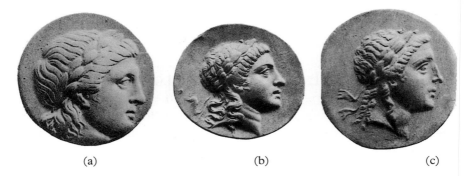

(a)   (b)   (c)

Figure 8
(a) Youthful head of Apollo with hair knotted on top and with a normal neck (from Myrina)
(b) Youthful head of Apollo with hair knotted at the nape of the neck and tumbling over his shoulders; the 'idealized neck' shows fat folds (from Myrina)
(c) Apollo with a goitre (from Myrina)
All three date to the second or first century BC. In the second century BC, the coin artists of Myrina portrayed anatomical variations of the neck. Their depiction of goitre suggests that the condition was endemic in the ancient world of the Mediterranean (BMC, M&W)

divination. Apollo was the presiding deity at the Delphic oracle in central Greece where the centre of the classical world was marked by a symbolic representation of the human navel or omphalos. A tripod or large serpent is also often seen on coins — the serpent represents Apollo slaying the python guarding the prophetic shrine of Apollo at Delphi (Figure 9b)[2]. The serpent-entwined staff was later acquired as an attribute of his medical role. His greatest medical feat was the relief of

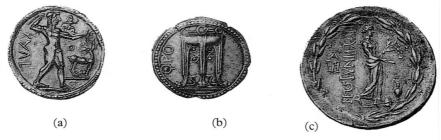

(a)   (b)   (c)

Figure 9   Other attributes of Apollo
(a) Coin from Caulonia depicting an 'archaic style' nude Apollo (c525–480 BC). The hunting role of Apollo is shown by the depiction of a stag and a ?sling (CNG)
(b) Coin from Croton (c510 BC) showing the Delphic tripod with three handles and legs terminating in lion's feet with serpents between (CNG)
(c) Coin from Myrina (165 BC) depicting Apollo holding a branch and a phiale with an omphalos and amphora at his feet (CNG)

the epidemic of Rome in 453 BC, for which he was honoured with the epithet 'Medicus'. Apollo was associated with many other activities and acquired several other epithets[3].

As Greek and Roman societies became more sophisticated, they developed a greater interest in health and longevity. Health matters needed to be separate from Apollo's other human endeavours, especially at temples dedicated to the hunt. Although his priests were elected officials without training, their duties reflected their personalities and interests. Priests at hunting shrines most likely had experience with hunting and probably did not possess the sensitivity needed for a medical role. In addition, such sanctuaries may well have lacked an ambience conducive to healing.

The need for a separate god of medicine was solved by the choice of mythological Apollo as the father of Asclepius. This achieved family continuity for medical care and also reflected the father-to-son tradition of Greek medical training. Asclepius' other qualifications for the role were impeccable. He had been born by Caesarean section and trained by Chiron. Asclepius and his serpents had chthonian associations and his medical skills surpassed those of Apollo while demonstrating his ability to raise the dead[4]. He survived punishment by Zeus, was raised to be the brightest star in the constellation of Scorpio, and was subsequently resurrected to become the god of medicine. The transfer of healthcare from Apollo to Asclepius was gradual. However, Asclepius was not accepted by the Gaulish peoples, for whom Apollo maintained the medical role[5]. Asclepius was introduced to mankind in a similar fashion to the present-day trial of a new doctor in a medical practice. He became a locum physician and underwent a probationary period in the practice to assess his skills and compatibility with patients and staff. He served initially at the temples of Apollo Maleatas, where the services to Apollo and Asclepius were joined. They shared the same temple and divided their sacrifices at Tricca and Epidaurus (fourth century BC) (ET 516), at Piraeus (355 BC) and at Athens where the sacrifices were also shared with the hunters and their dogs (ET 515). The transition period from Apollo to Asclepius can be traced numismatically. Asclepius' earliest known numismatic depiction is on a coin from Larissa, 450–400 BC (Figure 6b). This shows that he had, by then, become the predominant deity in that region of Thessaly but had not attained the stature of Apollo, whose help was sought in 453 BC to relieve the epidemic in Rome. After the Athenian defeat in the Peloponnesian War (431–404 BC), the Greeks sought the assistance of terrestrial gods, such as Asclepius, with whom they felt a closer and more sympathetic bond. This gave impetus to the acceptance of Asclepius and, as he grew in popularity, many of the temples of Apollo were re-dedicated to him. Thus, Corinth built an Asclepian temple on the site of its temple of Apollo[2]. Asclepius first appeared on the coins of Epidaurus in 370 BC, when he began to assume the senior medical role at its famous sanctuary of Apollo Maleatas. Apollo was still medically active in 323 BC (Figure 31a, chapter 4).

Asclepius was not universally accepted throughout the Graeco-Roman world. For instance, Julius Caesar regarded Apollo as the main healing deity of the Celtic tribes in Gaul, and archaeological evidence from Roman Britain suggests that Apollo was one of the healing deities worshipped by the native and Romano-British populations[6]. However, Asclepius was acknowledged by the Celtic tribes when they credited the origin of amber to 'the tears of Apollo', the very tears that had resulted from Apollo's grief at Zeus' execution of Asclepius by a thunderbolt (ET 110). Apollo retained his association with plague and pestilence and held senior consultant status with these diseases, thought to be associated with arrows strung from his bow as described in the *Iliad*. Furthermore, Apollo's later association with the sun and light, which now appears to be no earlier than the fifth century BC, led to crediting him with the invention of ophthalmology. He became consultant emeritus in this field of medicine.

Apollo and Asclepius adolescens

Apollo and Asclepius maintained close liaison. This is attested in Macrobius *Saturnalia*, written c400 AD: 'Asclepius is the same as Apollo' (ET 301), and by Eusebius who, in c300 AD, asked the question: 'How could the same be both father and son, Asclepius and at the same time Apollo?' *Praeparatio Evangelica*, III, 13, 15–16 (ET 298).

Calamis, an early fifth century BC Greek sculptor, depicted the gods in their youth; this tradition, however, was not continued in subsequent centuries. Some historians have interpreted the youthful depiction of Asclepius as symbolic of medical cure and the rejuvenation of an ailing body. Some ancient thinkers did not accept the artistic contrast of a contemporary youthful father (Apollo) and his middle-aged son (Asclepius). Cicero wrote in *The nature of the gods* (III 34, 83) (ET 683) that King Dionysius ordered the removal of Asclepius' golden beard from a statue at Syracuse as he did not think it appropriate for a son to wear a beard while his father did not. The apparent youthfulness of the father made it difficult to identify between Apollo and Asclepius and contributed to the formation of the term

'Asclepius adolescens'. This epithet was invented by recent historians to explain coins and statues showing a nude young man accompanied by a serpent-entwined staff. These statues portray a smooth and youthful face which was the antithesis of the kind, mature and bearded demeanour of Asclepius (Figure 4).

Warwick Wroth, the 19th century keeper of coins and medals in the British Museum, was the first to suggest that the depiction of a youthful figure holding a serpent-entwined staff represented Apollo and not Asclepius adolescens[7]. This conclusion was based on the similar appearance of the nude youth to the standard artistic depictions of Apollo. Even in ancient times, the nude sartorial habit of Apollo was an unacceptable dress code for a physician. Two coin types support Wroth's hypothesis. The first coin was minted at Lugdunum (Lyons), the capital of Gaul, in 70 or 71 AD in honour of the memory of the assassinated Emperor Galba — the first of four emperors who ruled Rome during 69 AD, the turbulent year of civil war following the suicide of Nero the previous year. This coin was minted by Vespasian, the last of these four emperors in power that year. The reverse of this coin depicts a standing, nude figure holding a serpent-entwined staff. Mattingly felt the standing figure represented Apollo or a local healing cult. Apollo Grannus was the most revered deity in Gaul and was the most appropriate god to be associated with this posthumous tribute to Emperor Galba. At the same time, the appearance of Apollo Grannus on the coin would acknowledge the loyalty of the Gauls. The addition of a serpent–staff symbol in his hand would have been acceptable to both the local population and the Senate and Rome population[8–10].

Mattingly's hypothesis is further supported by a major series of coins minted simultaneously in 207 AD by Emperor Severus and his joint successors, his sons, Geta and Caracalla. This issue coincides with the beginning of a definitive and massive expedition to reconsolidate their position in Britain. The obverse of the coins shows ruler portraits while the reverse depicts a nude, beardless youth whose right axilla rests on a long, serpent-entwined staff. This figure, flanked by two erect serpents, is standing on a podium in a bistyle (two-column) temple featuring a wreathed pediment and surmounting statues[10]. The nude figure in this historical setting is Apollo, not Asclepius adolescens, contrary to accepted, standard catalogue descriptions. Apollo is thought to be standing in the temple of Apollo Grannus in Gaul which today is located in the French village of Grand in the Vosges (Figure 10). The modern map confirms the existence of an early settlement at this site.

Three historical facts influence this interpretation. First, Apollo continued his medical role as both protector from and inflictor of

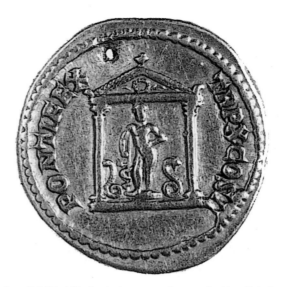

Figure 10 Coin of 207 AD depicting a nude youth (Apollo) holding a serpent-entwined staff and standing on a podium in a bistyle temple. The coin was perforated for suspension and used as a talisman (Photograph by the British Museum and reproduced with permission from the Trustees © Copyright The British Museum)

plague and pestilence. Second, Severus, Geta and Caracalla would have known of the disastrous effects of the plague of the Emperor Antoninus Pius' reign, which infected members of the victorious army of Avidius Cassius had carried back to Rome in 166 AD[11]. Deaths from the resulting epidemic extended throughout the Empire and the resulting mortality and confusion weakened the frontier defences of the Roman empire. The plague continued until 189 AD and included Emperor Marcus Aurelius (180 AD) among its victims. Undoubtedly, these three leaders did not wish an epidemic to make their expedition a repeat of the 163–4 AD 'Pyrrhic Roman victory in Parthia' when the troops brought back the most destructive plague in Roman history (Cary M 1954). The best prophylaxis against the pestilential arrows of Apollo would have been propitiation of the most powerful medical deity in the Western provinces of the empire by striking coins showing his portrait and his temple at Grand. Third, these coins also rendered symbolic recognition to the tribes of Gaul, whose capital had been ravaged by the forces of Severus during the civil war initiated by Clodius Albinus, Caesar of Britain, Spain and Gaul. This gesture of recognition would help secure Gallic loyalty and the army's essential supply route across the continent.

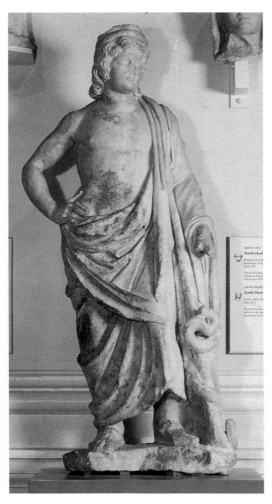

Figure 11 A larger than life-size statue of 'Asclepius adolescens' found at Cyrene. He has a youthful face and is wearing a *himation*; there is large serpent-entwined staff on the left (© Trustees of the National Museums of Scotland)

Some statues found at temples of Apollo, ie the temple of Apollo Maleatas at Epidaurus, portray a young man or adolescent dressed in the traditional Asclepian *himation* and holding a serpent-entwined staff. These depictions should be considered to represent Apollo. They denoted Apollo's retained medical role in Greek and Roman society; a statue in the British Museum depicts a clothed but 'flashing' Apollo accompanied by a lyre and serpent, indicating both his medical and musical roles. However, a similarly clothed adolescent, such as the ones from the temple of Asclepius at Epidaurus and Cyrene (Figure 11), represents a true Asclepius adolescens. This depiction symbolizes physical regeneration and rejuvenation similar to the serpent's annual shedding of its skin and medical healing of an ailing body.

The Vatican Museum exhibits the statue of a beardless Asclepius described as 'Asclepius adolescens' — the statue may have been ordered by Emperor Augustus to portray his personal physician, Antonius Musa.

> 'In honour of his physician, Antonius Musa, through whose care he [Augustus] had recovered from a critical illness; a sum of money was raised and Musa's statue set up alongside that of Asclepius.' (Suetonius, *Augustus*, 59) (ET 644)

This sculpture was executed in the likeness of Asclepius but portrays a beardless, 30-year-old man wearing the *himation* and supporting his right shoulder on a stout staff entwined by a large serpent. Musa was an Asclepiad, symbolized by his statue positioned next to Asclepius'. It is believed by the art historian, Schouten, that the Vatican Museum statue was based on one of Asclepius whose head had been altered to portray the distinguished physician[12].

In numismatic usage, the term 'Asclepius adolescens' should be abandoned and a youth, depicted nude and holding a serpent-entwined staff, should be identified as Apollo. However, at an Asclepian temple site, an adolescent shown wearing a *himation* and holding a serpent-entwined staff could symbolize Asclepius undergoing rejuvenation. In other settings, a similarly depicted beardless adult could be identified as an Asclepiad, while at certain locations, such as the temple of Apollo Maleatas, the younger person may also represent Apollo.

Prophecy and prognosis

Apollo was the god of prophecy and divination who foretold the outcome of future events, while Asclepius was the god of prognosis who predicted the outcome of illness.

Delphi was the chthonian centre *par excellence* which was protected by a large serpent called Python. In order to capture the site, Apollo killed the snake. He then appointed a priestess called the Pythia who sat concealed within the innermost sanctuary of the temple, wreathed in laurel leaves and seated on a tripod with serpent-entwined legs (Figure 9b). Shaking a laurel, the Pythia would issue her prophecies under divine inspiration, a state similar to a self-induced trance. She would utter obscure words and prophetic phrases which were interpreted by others in her retinue.

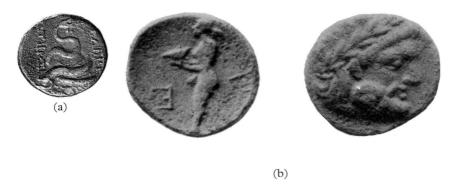

Figure 12
(a) Coin of Pergamum (133 BC–Augustus) depicting a netted omphalos encircled by a serpent and inscribed 'Asclepius the Saviour' (GDH)
(b) A husband and wife coin of Epidaurus (third or fourth century BC) depicting i) Epione on the reverse pouring from a vial into a patera and ii) Asclepius on the obverse (BMC, M&W)

Delphi became the foremost prophetic centre in the ancient world. Here, Apollo's priestesses made prophesies for a worldwide clientele of the rich and famous. Asclepius, on the other hand, limited his predictions to the outcome or prognosis of illness. The prognostic questions asked in those days still form a major component of current medical practice. Such questions include: will the patient recover? How long will recovery take? Will there be any residual disability? How long will the patient live?

The Delphic oracle supported Apollo's retirement from medical practice. In 292 BC, the Pythia referred a delegation of Roman politicians to Asclepius at Epidaurus, which resulted in the adoption of Asclepius into the Roman pantheon (see chapter 7). This initiated the spread of Asclepian worship throughout the ancient world.

The symbol for both prophecy and prognosis was the omphalos, a dome-shaped stone located at Delphi which represented the centre of the world[13]. The omphalos possessed a netlike pattern on its surface and was encircled by a large serpent representing either the Python of Apollo or the serpent of Asclepius (Figure 12a). Many coins of both Apollo and Asclepius depict the omphalos on the reverse, and Asclepian coins frequently associate his serpent with the symbol of prognosis and prophecy. A unique demonstration of the association of both Apollo and Asclepius with a serpent-entwined omphalos is provided on the coin minted in 244 AD by Philippus Senior, commemorating the myth of Asclepius (Figure 7).

The divine retinue — Asclepius and his family

Asclepius delegated aspects of healthcare to various members of his family who worked under his direction as auxiliary divinities. His wife, Epione, played an active role in the early days of Asclepian temple medicine. Her role was similar to the traditional role of doctors' spouses, assisting in the establishment of a medical practice. Asclepius is credited with fathering a number of children, although the precise number is not clear. His sons, including Machaon, Podalirius, Ianiscus (healer), Euemerion or, in Doric dialect, Euamerion (good health) and Acesis (healing) were part of the divine healthcare team as were his daughters including Hygieia, Panacea, Aegle (radiance) and, the more obscure personifications of words for healing, Iaso and Aceso.

Epione

Epione was Heracles' daughter (Hippocrates, ET 162) and her name, according to Cornutus, indicates 'the relief of complaints with the help of soothing medicines' (ET 281). Her duties are thought to have involved preparing and administrating medicines, as shown on a coin of the third or fourth century BC from Epidaurus which carries a depiction of her pouring from a vial into a *patera* (dish) (Figure 12b). Two statues of Epione at Epidaurus reflect an ancient counterpart of 'town and gown': one was located in the town and the other in the temple precinct. As the family expanded in size, Epione became less involved with medical care and her children followed the Greek tradition of entering their father's trade.

Machaon

Machaon was an Homeric hero who, with Podalirius, preceded the creation of the Asclepian myth. In the *Iliad*, Machaon was a surgeon and a soldier. He became famous after treating the Greek expeditionary leader Menelaus' wound (ET 164) and later became the patron of surgeons. According to Quintus of Smyrna, Machaon was one of the Greek heroes who entered Troy hidden in the wooden horse, but died in the subsequent fighting from a wound made by a three-barbed arrow in the shoulder. He was given a hero's tomb in the Messenian city of Gerenia. His sons, Alexenor and Sphyrus, founded the Asclepieia at Titane in Sicyon and in Argos respectively.

Podalirius

Podalirius was also a physician and soldier at Troy. He is hardly mentioned by Homer in the *Iliad*, but post-Homeric writers have exaggerated his presence at Troy, giving him equal or greater status

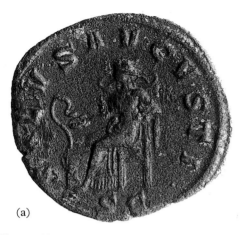
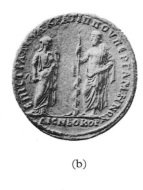

(b)

(a)

Figure 13
(a) Hygieia feeding an erect serpent from a *patera* depicted on a Sestertius of Maximinus. The inscription reads '*Salus Augusti*' (Health to the emperors) (GDH)
(b) Coin from Pergamum during the reign of L. Verus (161–9 AD) depicting Asclepius with a tall staff encircled by a serpent in his right hand; he faces Hygieia, who is wearing a *chiton*, *peplos* and veil, and who is standing on his right holding a serpent in her right hand (BMC, M&W)

than Machaon. Podalirius gained medical fame for his skills in treating internal diseases after he was said to have diagnosed and cured Ajax's madness, and had used a salve provided by his father to heal the wounds of two warriors (ET 199). After the Greek victory, Podalirius went to Italy where he married and had two children. There is no record of his family continuing the tradition of medical practice.

Ianiscus, Euemerion and Acesis
Ianiscus appeared as a naked youth on a coin of Bizye but little else is recorded about him. Pausanias stated that Euemerion was recognized at the Asclepieion at Titane where his statue was paired with Alexenor, and that Pergamenes identified Euemerion with Telesphorus while Epidaurians called him Acesis (ET 749). Ianiscus and Acesis did not participate in Asclepian temple medicine.

Hygieia
Hygieia became a partner in the practice of Asclepian temple medicine and achieved full divinity. Her role as the goddess of health has survived to the present-day in the modern medical terminology of hygiene and hygienic. The importance of her role is indicated by many statues and coin portraits that show her to be an attractive, young, professional woman wearing a veil and a *chiton* or *peplos* (rectangular

piece of cloth fastened at each shoulder). She was usually depicted holding either a *patera* or a sacred serpent (Figures 13a, 18). The *patera* contained either food for the serpent or the elixir of life for man. A combined portrait of her with Asclepius symbolized the treatment of illness and the return to health (Figure 13b). Her Roman name was Salus and, in Roman times, her role expanded to include protecting the emperor's and state's health. Almost every emperor minted a coin with her depiction and the inscription '*Salus Augusti*' (health and safety of the emperor) or '*Salus Publica*' (safety of the state) — despite this added political role, she was always accompanied by an Asclepian serpent.

In the first century BC, the Romans also linked her with Valetudo, their deity associated with convalescence and who gave rise to the word *valetudinarium* (military hospital). The highest mark of respect for Salus was shown on an inscription found in the Roman fort at Caerleon, Wales, which carried the epithet 'regina' (queen). The Romans were not rigid in their name for the goddess of health; Minerva, the Roman equivalent for the Greek goddess Athena, sometimes replaced or substituted for Salus and, on these occasions, became Minerva Medica. The practice of associating Minerva with Salus originated both in Athens, where there stood an altar to Hygieia-Athena as well as statues to Athene also named Hygieia[12], and at the Asclepieion of Epidaurus, where there was a large statue of Athena holding a serpent-entwined staff of Asclepius. Sometimes, Roman portraits of Salus were copied from Minerva or Minerva Medica from Salus. In these circumstances, the Athenian helmet was omitted and Athena's serpent, Erichthonius, was replaced by the Asclepian serpent[14]. An interesting example of the overlap between Minerva and Salus was found at Coventina's Well on Hadrian's Wall. Here, a statue depicting Minerva standing on the right of Asclepius was found (Figure 14). The Roman practice of assigning a Roman name to a foreign deity with similar interests and then adopting that deity occurred in the case of the celestial Celtic goddess Brigantia, who became associated with Salus at Corbridge[15].

Hygieia has occasionally been described as Asclepius' wife. This error probably originated with 'Hymn 57 of Orpheus' which contained the words: 'All-healing Asclepius, ... you who have as your wife, faultless Hygieia' *Orphei Hymni*, LXVII (ET 601). Further substance has been provided by some very attractive, artistic depictions displaying on occasion overt affection between the two. These include the coin from Bizya, Thrace (BMC), which depicts Asclepius reclining on a couch with his hand on Hygieia's shoulder, and the antique

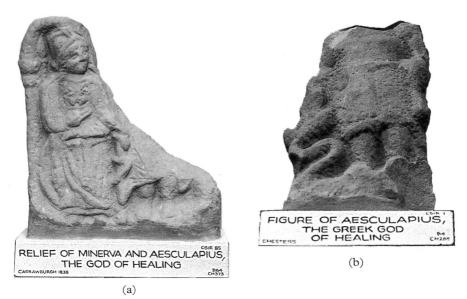

Figure 14
(a) Statue (second century AD) from Coventina's Well, Hadrian's Wall, which portrays Minerva standing on the right of a mutilated Asclepius (32.5 cm×30 cm)
(b) This statue, displayed next to (a) by the Chesters Museum, is another mutilated Asclepius, found at the fort of Cilurnum (Chesters), Hadrian's Wall
(Photo GDH; courtesy of Dr Grace Simpson, curator, Chesters Museum, Hadrian's Wall Museums, England)

marble in the Vatican Museum portraying Hygieia and Asclepius seated on a couch. The latter shows her right hand on Asclepius' shoulder and her *chiton* unfastened, exposing her right breast. However, the relationship is correct on the coins of Epidaurus which show Epione with Asclepius (323–240 BC) (Figure 12b).

Panacea
Panacea has been described as having a name derived from the Greek word 'acos' (remedy), thus implying medical treatment. She does not seem to have played a major role in temple medical practice, but her name was included in the oath of Hippocrates and is the derivation of the modern English word 'panacea' which means a cure-all.

Iaso and Aceso
Iaso and Aceso did not have significant roles in Asclepian medical practice. Iaso's name derived from the Greek verb *iasthai* meaning 'to heal'. Little is mentioned of these two daughters except in an inscription (*Inscriptiones Graecae* II, No 4962) (ET 515) written in

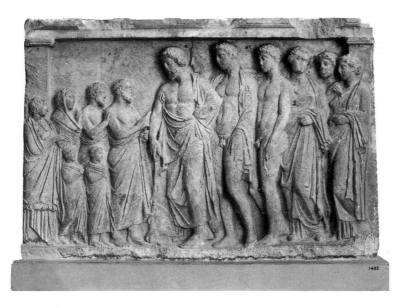

Figure 15 The divine retinue: Asclepius resting on a crutch-like staff, Hygieia, Machaon, Podalirius, Panacea, Aceso and Iaso. Votive relief from Thyrea in Argolis c370–360 BC (Photo © National Archaeological Museum of Greece, Athens)

the fourth century BC. This described the temple ritual in which the two daughters, along with Maleas, Apollo, Hermes, Panacea, the dogs and the huntsmen, each receive three sacrificial cakes as part of the initial ritual. Interestingly, Asclepius himself is not mentioned (it is to be hoped they saved some for him!).

Scholarly marginal comments on Aristophanes' early fourth century BC play, *Plutus*, mention another daughter Aegle (ET 278 & 279) who is also referred to in other classical sources (eg, the Elder Pliny). Asclepius' mother, Coronis, may have been used as a fertility talisman. In addition to the coin shown in Figure 3, there were some statues of her and one, found near the temple of Sulis Minerva at Bath, may indicate a possible association of Asclepius with the temple of Sulis Minerva.

Asclepius and his family of auxiliary divinities consulting with a patient and his family are shown in Figure 15. On this bas-relief from Thyrea in Argolis dated c370–360 BC, Machaon and Podalirius are depicted nude. Nudity was the traditional presentation for Greek hero-gods and this depiction was created at a time when Asclepius had a major following for a hero-god status. That Asclepius was usually depicted clothed may reflect patient preference (we expect the consultants of today to be conservatively attired). In this sculpture, the greater status of the gods is emphasized by the six deities who tower above the patient and his family. Today's counterpart of this sculpture would be professorial rounds in a teaching hospital, where members of the healthcare team assemble around the bedside and tower, like gods, above the patient while they discuss the case.

Telesphorus

Later, Telesphorus (accomplisher) was also considered a son, perhaps synonymous with Acesis[12]. The Athenians considered Telesphorus to be the third son of Asclepius but he was not depicted on the fourth century BC relief from Thyrea (Figure 15). His earliest Athenian reference was 190–200 AD in *Inscriptiones Graecae* III (ET 287), which credits him with saving Athens from an epidemic. Telesphorus was a separate god with his own followers but, over time, he became closely associated with Asclepius. He became the Greek god of convalescence, and may have been the divinity associated with sleep, perfect health, magical healing and even blood letting. Although junior to Asclepius, he supplied disciplines previously missing from the divine healthcare team and was evoked separately to 'restore to full health the person who is ready to receive him' (ET 313). He was depicted as a small figure clothed in a hooded cape (Figure 16) and his arms muffled in his mantle. This attire may have been the garb of an ambulatory patient with a fever, or a convalescent, and is not unlike some of today's dressing gowns. Alternatively, it may have been a simple night gown worn by people confined to bed or about to undergo temple sleep. The hooded cape has also been described as a symbol of magic medicine and is reminiscent of that worn by a wizard. There is an interesting resemblance between this figure and the *genii cucullati* of the Celts, whose *cucullus* was a large, hooded cape covering the shoulders or a cloak over the whole body to the knees [personal

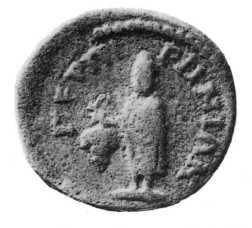

Figure 16   Bronze coin (138–61 AD) depicting Telesphorus on the reverse wearing hooded garb of a convalescent and holding a bunch of grapes. Coins from Perperene in Mysia portray on their reverse a bunch of grapes as their identifying symbol. Their association with Telesphorus may have been an advertisement for the convalescent properties of the regional wines (BMC, M&W)

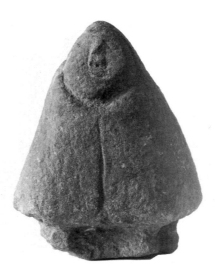

Figure 17 Statue of Telesphorus from Birdoswald fort on Hadrian's Wall, dating to the second or third century AD (height c45 cm) (© Tullie House City Museum and Art Gallery, Carlisle, England)

communication: R Brickstock][16,17]. These gods usually appeared in threes, in Celtic custom a device used to increase the power of these small deities. A statue of Telesphorus was found at the Roman fort of Birdoswald on Hadrian's Wall (Figure 17). The similarity of a *genius cucullatus* to Telesphorus is such that the museum at Carlisle has one such figure labelled 'Telesphorus or Cucullatus'.

Hadrian (117–138 AD) was the first emperor to depict Telesphorus on coins, a practice continued by Emperors Antoninus Pius, Commodus, Trajan, Caracalla and others; the coins were minted in the Greek-speaking, eastern provinces of the Roman empire at cities with an Asclepian temple[17,18,21]. Telesphorus was depicted frequently with Hygieia, Asclepius and their serpents. When this medical triumvirate appeared on a coin, it may have been a thanks offering for treatment (Figure 18).

Telesphorus could have originated from a *genius cucullatus* brought into Asia Minor with the Celtic invasion of 278 BC. These Celtic tribes, serving as mercenaries for Nicomedes of Bythinia and Mithridates of Pontus, were employed to plunder the lands to the south belonging to the Seleucid King Antiochus. The Celts settled in Galatia and continued to raid Seleucid territory but were finally attacked and defeated by the forces of Pergamum in 179 BC. During this conflict, Pergamum captured 40,000 prisoners and celebrated the victory by building an altar to Zeus, decorated with a marble relief to

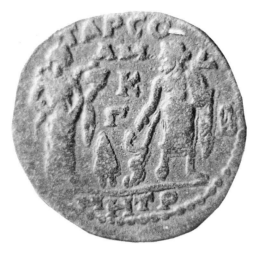

Figure 18 Coin of Maximinus I (235–8 AD) from Tarsus (Cilicia) depicting Asclepius with staff and serpent in his right hand, Hygieia standing on his right holding and feeding a large rigid serpent, and with Telesphorus standing between them. The depiction of this medical 'triumvirate' often reflected the emperor recovering from illness (GDH)

commemorate the defeat of the Celts[22]. It is possible that veneration of a Celtic *cucullatus* was introduced into Asia Minor at that time and a medical deity evolved. The god's acceptance by Pergamum could explain the first numismatic depiction of Telesphorus on their coins. These coins help clarify the previously tenuous link between the *cucullatus* of the Celts and the Graeco-Roman Telesphorus. On the other hand, a coin minted by the Gaulish Segusiavi (58–27 BC) is considered by some to be a representation of Telesphorus himself[14]. Perhaps this orphan, Celtic god became Asclepius' adopted son!

A third century AD hymn to Telesphorus stated that he was celebrated at Athens but worshipped as Acesis at Epidaurus.

Asclepiads

The term 'Asclepiad' was applied to physicians of ancient Greece. It derived from the ancient Greek word 'Asclepiadae' which literally translated means the offspring of Asclepius. There is uncertainty about its origin. One view suggests that there was an ancient clan of hereditary physicians who claimed to have descended from Asclepius. Aelius Aristides supported this view in the second century AD in *Oratio* XXXVIII (ET 282), by describing Machaon and Podalirius as the first Asclepiads to settle in Cos and there founded a medical dynasty.

Another view, now discarded, was that the Asclepiadae were the early priest-physicians of the Asclepian temples. This theory incorrectly implied that Hippocratic medicine evolved directly from temple medicine.

There may be a practical explanation for the origin of the term, namely the earliest Greek physicians were itinerant artisans who peddled their trade from village to village and sought patients wherever people congregated, notably at markets, temples and festivals. They were also guests of various households in need of medical services, for which they received shelter and a place to pray. In the fifth century BC, no laws existed to protect persons away from their homes; in order to protect themselves, physicians banded together to form the first association of craftsmen which was the forerunner of medieval guilds and present-day medical associations. This association also served the teaching of their craft by apprenticeship with a strong father-to-son tradition but did not totally exclude others. The apprenticeship system had no clear-cut line separating qualified from unqualified; the criteria were probably the degree of usefulness and the willingness to continue in the subservient role of an apprentice. Qualification may also have been influenced by the time of indenture agreed on at the beginning of the training period.

Although this association of craftsmen used the term Asclepiad, they did not claim to be descended from Asclepius. Their choice of name implying son of their patron god had its equivalent with the Homeridae, a guild devoted to the recitation of the Homeric poems, which flourished in the island of Chios. They did not claim to be blood-descendants of Homer; similarly, artists became Daedalidae after Daedalus and early pharmacists, who had learnt the skills of Chiron, became Chironidae.

The earliest literary reference to the Asclepiads appears in a sarcastic reference to their potential of acquiring wealth from medical practice in the poetry of Theognis of Megara (ET 219), who is believed to have lived in the seventh century BC:

> 'If god had granted it to the Asclepiads, to heal evil deeds and the hearts of those who are blinded by reckless actions, they would earn great amounts of money'.

The best definition of Asclepiad appears in the 12th century *Book of histories*, written by the Byzantine poet Ioannes Tzetzes in *Chiliades* XII, 637–39 (ET 228). This author produced a hypothetical contemporary letter describing the status of the Asclepiads in classical Greece: 'Normally speaking, Asclepiads are those who are descended from the offspring of Asclepius. But now, through misuse, the term has come to mean physicians'. It is likely that Tzetzes was able to study ancient texts no longer available to present-day historians and that its use in ancient Greece was certainly synonymous with physician (*iatros*). Its use is now considered archaic; the word did not become Romanized but was replaced by the Latin *medicus*.

Hippocrates

Hippocrates is the most famous Asclepiad, recognized today as the father of clinical medicine. Plato (427–348/7 BC) referred to him in his dialogue, *Phaedrus*, as the 'Asclepiad' (ET 217) and Aristotle designated him as 'leader of the Asclepiads' (ET 218). He was born on the island of Cos in 460 or 459 BC and studied medicine at Cos, Ionia, Egypt and Asia. As a physician, he travelled and taught far and wide. He was consulted by the rich and famous, including King Perdiccas of Macedon and Ataxerxes of Persia.

Hippocrates also studied philosophy at many famous centres in the ancient world. At Ephesus, he studied the papyri on natural phenomena donated by Heraclitus and, at Miletus, met the philosopher Anaxagoras who taught him the theory of matter. At Samos, the philosopher Melissus taught him the theories of Pythagoras.

From his broad background of learning and clinical experience, Hippocrates devised a concept of illness. He removed it from the realms of superstition and based it on natural causes. His treatise on the 'sacred disease' (epilepsy) began with: 'It is not, in my opinion, any more sacred than other diseases, but it has a natural cause and its supposed divine origin is due to people's inexperience and to their amazement at its unusual character'[23]. The discussion went on to elaborate the Hippocratic concept of disease and physical causes, but its anatomical and physiological foundations were weak and details of the Hippocratic discourse were erroneous.

Hippocrates based the aetiology of disease on an imbalance of physical forces which incorporated the basic elements and qualities of the universe: fire (hot), air (cold), earth (dry) and water (moist). These, in turn, were represented in the body by four humours: black bile, yellow bile, phlegm and blood. Health was a state of harmonious mixture of the humours; sickness occurred when an excess or deficiency of certain external and internal factors resulted in an imbalance of the body humours. Treatment, such as that involving diet, fluids, purging or bleeding, was aimed at restoring this imbalance (see chapter 8).

Hippocrates' thoughts and those of the Hippocratic doctors are known from *The Hippocratic corpus*, a compilation of about 70 treatises,

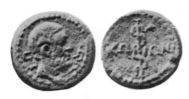

Figure 19 The obverse of a coin from Cos (second century AD) depicting Hippocrates. The reverse of the coin shows Asclepius' staff (BMC, M&W)

written in the fifth and fourth centuries BC — they were collated in Alexandria c280 BC. Modern scholars have studied these and concluded that he was not actually the author of the writings bearing his name. Jones, translator of *Hippocrates* volumes I, II and IV (1923–31) stated that 'of the roughly seventy works in the Hippocratic Collection many are not by Hippocrates; even the famous oath may not be his. That he was the Father of Medicine no one should deny.'[24]. The contemporary Canadian historian, Dr Potter, who translated volumes V, VI and VIII of *The Hippocratic corpus* in the 1980s, repeated these words but added: 'the corpus is likely to have originated in the school of Hippocrates on Cos'[25].

These texts cover a variety of subjects that Jones and Potter have examined in detail. They contained much teaching material that would have been used at the Coan Medical School. The oath of Hippocrates and some of the ethical descriptions of the writings are outlined in chapter 7, along with aspects of prognosis and clinical description. For further information, readers are referred to the work and translations of Jones and Potter, and the other volumes in the Loeb Classical Library.

Hippocrates' portrait has survived on ancient coins. Two of these are extremely rare and are considered to be contemporary portraits. The best known is a second century AD coin from the island of Cos. This shows Hippocrates to be bald, with prominent eyes and a beard (Figure 19). These features are also displayed on a Roman copy of a Hellenistic bust found at Ostia Antica, the ancient port of Rome, and on a late Hellenistic portrait discovered on Cos[26]. Hippocrates is believed to have lived for more than 100 years and is thought to have been buried at Larissa in Thessaly, northern Greece, the area in which Asclepius was said to have been brought up. He continues to live in the minds of physicians. The International Hippocratic Foundation of Cos was founded in 1960 to cultivate for today's world the conscience and ideal of medicine conceived and applied by this most renowned Asclepiad.

Notes and references

1. The first Greek physician to the gods was Paeon. His name first appears on the Cnossus Tablets from late Bronze Age Crete. 'Io Paeon' was used in the hymn of invocation to Apollo and, later, title was applied to Asclepius and other deities. The word came to mean a song of praise or thanksgiving and a shout of triumph.

2. Lang M. *Cure and cult in ancient Corinth. American excavations in old Corinth. Corinth notes no 1*. American School of Classical Studies at Athens, 1977.

3. Maleatas was an archaic healing and hunting deity at Epidaurus. Apollo became associated with him and acquired his name. Other epithets of Apollo include: 'Cyparissius' which referred to the holy cypress grove on the island of Cos where Hippocrates stated that the assumption of the staff was celebrated (ET 568); 'Smintheus', Greek for mouse and associated with famine and plague. In the *Iliad*, Apollo was associated with both bringing and relieving the plague; 'Hecatebolus' referred to his power to administer sudden death as with the Cyclops and the plague; 'Alexicacus' was a name for a healer-god who drove away illness; 'Lucoctone' was the killer of wolves; 'Musagetes', meaning accompanied by the muses referred to Apollo's musical talents. 'Parnopais' (locust killer); 'Xanthus' fair; 'Chrysocomes' golden locks; 'Phoebus' brilliant; 'Lycian' light and 'Granno' shining. Most of the Greek epithets were descriptive whereas the Roman ones combined Apollo with the name of a foreign deity. Epithets of Asclepius are given in chapter 9.

4. Chthonian: underground and underworld. The realm of the old underground deities.

5. Wiseman A, Wiseman P. *Julius Caesar. The battle for Gaul: a new translation*. London: Chatto & Windus, 1980.

6. Excavations at Nettleton revealed a circular pit (18 feet diameter) thought to be associated with a ritual purpose similar to the tholos or snake-pit within the sanctuary of Asclepius at Epidaurus and the sanctuary of Apollo at Curium, Cypress. Wedlake WJ. *The excavation of the shrine of Apollo at Nettleton, Wiltshire, 1956–71*. The Society of Antiquaries, Thames and Hudson Ltd, 1982. Unfortunately, this excavation report does not mention a search for snake vertebrae that might remain at archaeological sites associated with snake pits.

7. Wroth W. *Apollo and the staff of Aesculapius*. NC vol II, 3rd series. 1882: 301–5.

8. Mattingly H. *Coins of the Roman empire in the British Museum*. Vol 1. London: Trustees of the British Museum, 1923 (reprinted 1965).

9. Mattingly H. *Coins of the Roman empire in the British Museum*. Vol 5. London: Trustees of the British Museum, 1950.

10. Mattingly H and Sydenham. *RIC IV* Part 1. London: Spink & Son, 1931.

11. The plague of Antoninus was also known as the plague of Galen. He wrote a brief description of the plague and fled Rome to avoid becoming a victim. Cartwright felt his flight set a precedent followed by London physicians during the Great Plague of 1665. Cartwright FF. Pandemics, past and future. In: Hart G, Irwin C, eds. *Disease in ancient man*. Toronto: Clark Iwin Inc, 1983: 267–80.

12. Schouten JS. *The rod and serpent of Asklepios*. New York: Elsevier Publishing Company, 1967.

13. Delphi was established as the centre of the earth by the meeting there of two eagles set free from the ends of the earth. This legend was illustrated by a coin showing two eagles sitting on the omphalos.

14. Storer HR. *Medicina in nummis*. Boston: Wright Potter Printing Co, 1931.

15. Birley E. *Corbridge Roman station*. London: HMSO, 1954.

16. The British equivalent was the *birrus Britannicus*, a hooded cloak of goat's hair which was one of the leading exports of the day.

17. Darenberg and Saglio. *Dictionaire des antiquities, Greques et Romaines*. Vol 5. Paris, 1877.

18. The existence of a separate but complementary cult dedicated to Telesphorus, first celebrated numismatically by Emperor Hadrian, may explain the execution

and martyrdom of the eighth Bishop of Rome whose name was also Telesphorus. If the Bishop had preached to his congregation condemning his pagan namesake, then Hadrian may have felt that this was sedition and acted accordingly. The Bishop was eventually canonized and became St Telesphore; standard references describing saints of the Roman Catholic Church neither mention his pagan namesake nor give a reason for his execution[19,20]. His martyrdom is still remembered in the province of Quebec, Canada, where there is a village and a church named after him. (Not too many motorists speeding along the MacDonald-Cartier Freeway linking Toronto with Montreal think of Hadrian, Pergamum and Asclepius when they pass the sign shown in Figure 20).

19. Baring-Gould S. *The lives of the saints*. Volume 1. Edinburgh: John Grant, 1914: 65.
20. Eric J. *The Popes: a concise biographical history*. London: Burns and Oates, 1964.
21. Wroth W. *J Hellenic Studies* 1882; **3**: 283–300. This emphasizes the numismatic sources for the study of Telesphorus and lists 17 cities in the western Mediterranean world that depicted Telesphorus on their coins. It also cites his depiction on a marble relief at Imbros in the islands of the Thracian Sea and an inscription to him, Hygieia and Asclepius from Verona.
22. MacCana P. *Celtic mythology*. London: The Hamlyn Publishing Group, 1970.
23. Goold GP, ed. The sacred disease. In: *Hippocrates*. Vol II translated by Jones WHJ. Loeb Classical Library. Massachusetts: Harvard University Press and London: William Heinemann Ltd. Reprinted 1992: 139.
24. Goold GP, ed. *Hippocrates*. Vols *I, II, IV* translated by Jones WHJ. Loeb Classical Library. Massachusetts: Harvard University Press and London: William Heinemann Ltd. Reprinted, vol I 1984, vol II 1992, vol IV 1992.
25. Goold GP, ed. *Hippocrates*. Vols *V, VI* translated by Potter P. Loeb Classic Library Massachusetts: Harvard University Press and London: William Heinemann Ltd, 1988.
26. Hart GD. Letter 'Authentic Hippocrates' with editor's reply. *Humane Medicine* 1994, **10**(1).

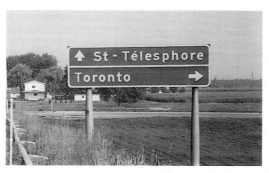

Figure 20 Telesphorus remembered in the Canadian province of Quebec: a current road sign on Highway 401, pointing to St Télesphore (GDH)

Chapter 3

Serpents, superstition and the gods

People in ancient times believed that the gods had bestowed special favour on serpents. The annual shedding of serpent skin symbolized the casting off of death, or the recovery from illness, followed by rebirth and regeneration. It was commonly thought that serpent tunnels were an entry to the underworld, providing access to the subterranean gods, and that they were able to contact the dead. The ability of serpents to form their bodies into a circle was regarded as a symbol of eternity and their absence of visible genitalia as a sign of supreme, procreative powers. It was thought that their keen vision was an indication of caution and wisdom and they believed that their vision coupled with their absence of sleep endowed them with extreme powers of vigilance. They marvelled at the serpent's ability to ingest prey with a greater body circumference than their own and it was believed that serpents acquired a special vital force from drinking milk. They feared the suffering and death resulting from the bite of a small adder. Finally, they believed that serpents had learned the medicinal powers of plants and herbs from their habitat among bushes. These beliefs resulted in association of the serpent with the healing deities of the Egyptians, Chaldeans and Semites, as well as the Greeks and Romans.

In addition to their connection with Asclepius, serpents were associated with many other Graeco-Roman deities. Athena wore a serpent emblem on her helmet and she also wore the *aegis* — a large bib with scales, fringed with serpents' heads and decorated with the snake-haired Gorgon. The Athenian hero, Erichthonius, adopted by Athena as her son and associated with her cult on the Acropolis, was sometimes made manifest in the form of a serpent. Apollo maintained an association with serpents via the Delphic oracle where he is said to have slain the giant serpent and to have seized the oracular shrine from Mother Earth. Hermes carried a wand or caduceus (the herald's symbol) which portrayed two intertwined serpents — this became the symbol of communication, peace and commerce. Serpents were also associated with the Greek gods (and their Roman equivalents), including: Zeus, Hera, Demeter, Dionysus, Persephone, Hecate (a goddess related to magic and witchcraft), and the protector god, Agathodaemon or Agathos Daemon, the god of good fortune to whom

41

the Greeks 'raised their wine glasses'. They were also associated with the Roman personifications of Felicitas (good fortune), Securitas, Fortuna, Concordia and Pax (peace). These beliefs reflected profound respect for the serpent, which became a symbol of life itself. In fact, serpents were worshipped for their versatile powers and the early practice of ophiolatry (serpent worship) is widely attested throughout the world. People from countries that do not have indigenous serpents, such as New Zealand, worshipped its aquatic counterpart, the eel[1].

Asclepius and serpents

Chapter 1 described how serpents guarded the infant Asclepius on Mount Pelion and taught him the medicinal properties of plants and herbs. His association with them continued and eventually evolved into one of metamorphosis, where Asclepius could change into a serpent and a serpent into Asclepius. Serpents played an integral role in the incubation ritual of Asclepian temple medicine and a temple serpent, brought from Epidaurus as the embodiment of Asclepius, was needed for the establishment of any new sanctuary. The 'Asclepian serpent' is considered by herpetologists to be *Elaphe longissima*, a snake of the family Colubridae. This species has been known to grow to a length of 200 cm (80 inches), but is usually < 140 cm (56 inches), averaging 1 cm diameter and 3.1 cm circumference. Ancient coins depicted its large size and frequently portrayed it rearing and holding itself erect (Figure 13a). It moves with great speed and, when approached, sometimes holds its ground while its jaws make chewing movements [personal communication: Savage HG, University of Toronto][2]. The species is a very adept climber and can ascend vertical tree trunks where it coils around branches waiting and watching for prey (Figures 21 & 22). Its diet consists mainly of small mammals and nestling birds. In spite of its great size, it is harmless to humans and may be treated as a domestic pet, a trait also demonstrated by an ancient coin portraying Valetudo or Salus allowing a large serpent to approach her mouth (Figure 56b).

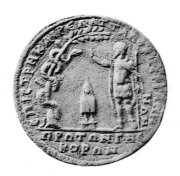

Figure 21 Coin of Pergamum (54 BC) showing the Asclepian serpent entwined around a tree trunk and being saluted by Emperor Caracalla, with a statue of Telesphorus in the centre (BMC, M&W)

Statues of Asclepius confirm the great length of the serpent and indicate a circumference greater

(a)

(b)

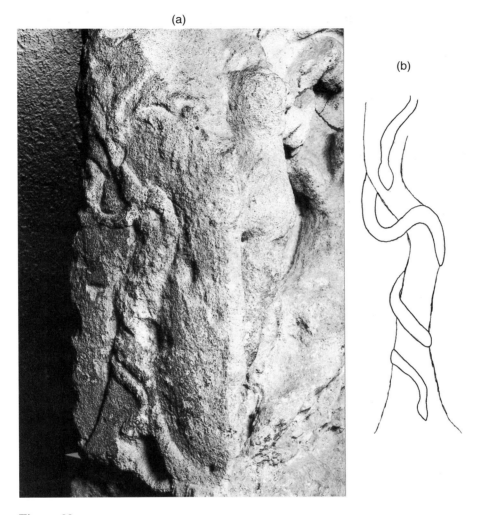

Figure 22
(a) A serpent encircling a branch of a tree depicted on an eroded bas-relief found at Bath, England. The front of this carving depicts Coronis and Apollo; the well preserved reverse depicts a small dog (courtesy of Ms Jane Bircher and the Roman Baths Museum, Bath, England)
(b) Drawing of serpent in Figure 22a, by Ms Cindy Buhle, Bracebridge, ON Canada

than today's average 3.1 cm. Ancient artists portrayed accurate details of proportion and the discrepancy in body diameter may be explained by the ancient requirement that only a serpent from Epidaurus could be used in the establishment of a new sanctuary. Had the Epidaurians learnt the technique of selective breeding, with the result that their serpents were significantly larger than those from other places? Or was the large girth a result of diet? Food was probably more plentiful at the temples than in the wild and perhaps serpent circumference was a reflection of caloric intake, just like a modern fat cat.

The present distribution of *Elaphe longissima* follows the boundaries of the Roman empire at the time of Julius Caesar, except that it only occurs in small, discrete areas in the north of Spain and the centre of Germany. Laughlin hypothesized that its current geographical distribution is a result of Asclepian temple abandonment, which led to the sacred serpents wandering out to live in the wild[3]. His suggestion is supported by the species habituating ruins and old walls, and by its curiously isolated populations in Switzerland and Germany, areas bordering Roman archaeological sites[4].

Another Elaphe species, *E. quattuorlineata*, resembles *E. longissima* but can reach greater length (up to 250 cm or 8 feet 4 inches) and is slightly broader (4 cm average diameter) — it is more phlegmatic and moves more slowly. Its present-day distribution is Italy and the coastal areas of Greece and the Aegean.

Asclepius' choice of *E. longissima* represented divine serendipity because its appetite for rodents would have kept temple compounds free of plague-transmitting rats and mice most effectively. Temple serpents also participated in the healing ritual and their saliva may have contained antiseptic properties. Italian doctors have recently demonstrated the presence of a growth factor and receptor in the oral, salivary and upper digestive epithelia of *E. quattuorlineata*. This suggests a convincing physiological basis for the reputed healing properties of a lick from an Asclepian snake[5]. An inscription on Stele I at Epidaurus describes the story of a man with a malignant sore on his toe who was cured by the tongue of a snake in the *abaton* (ET 423, *Inscriptiones Graecae* IV, 1, 121–22).

Serpent symbol of Asclepius

Asclepius is symbolized by a single serpent entwined around a staff — this was adopted by the Asclepiads. It was also used as a healing talisman as demonstrated by the small figure of Aesculapius found at Chichester, England. The surface of its serpent and staff symbol has been worn smooth and has become indistinct from frequent rubbing (Figure 23). The symbol almost disappeared after the establishment of Christianity and fall of Paganism. However, it was remembered on Greek and Roman coins which continued to circulate for many hundreds of years, and also in Rome where it was depicted on the portside of the marble ship prow which stood below the church of Saint Bartolomeo della Isola. A similar symbol was used in Christianity to depict Moses' relief of the plague of serpents by

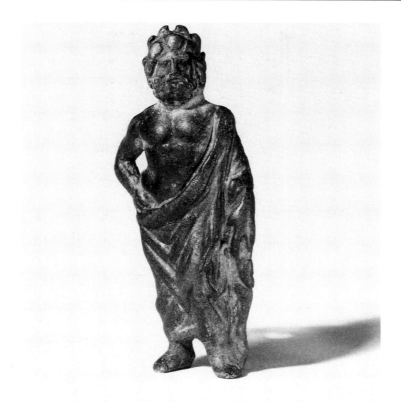

Figure 23 Bronze figurine of Aesculapius found at Chichester, West Sussex (64.1 mm high). Note that details of the staff and serpent are no longer distinct, probably as a result of wear caused by frequent supplications (© Copyright The British Museum and reproduced by permission of the Trustees)

erecting a brazen serpent on a staff. During the Renaissance in the 16th century, the Aesculapius symbol was rediscovered and restored to physicians. It was quickly accepted due to its similarity with the serpent of Moses, and is now incorporated in the heraldic crests of almost all National Medical Societies in the world (chapter 12). The activities of the World Health Organization (WHO) are carried out under this ancient banner, with the result that it has again acquired international meaning and symbolism. The WHO crest is almost an exact copy of the reverse of a Coan coin from the first century BC (Figure 24).

The staff of Asclepius may have originated with early Greek doctors travelling from village to village in search of patients. The roads were rough and lonely, so the stout staff served as a walking stick as well as a means of defence. It became a symbol of physicians, similar to the gold-headed cane of the 18th and 19th centuries.

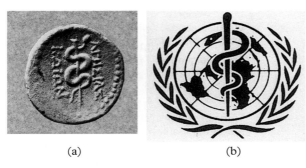

(a)   (b)

Figure 24 (a) Bronze coin of Cos (88–50 BC) depicting Asclepius on the obverse and his staff on the reverse (BMC, M&W)
(b) World Health Organization logo

The staff on coins and statuary was shown to be either short and held by the hand, or long and resting in the axilla as a crutch. Asclepius, or the artists depicting him, was probably ambidextrous as, although the staff was usually shown to be held in the right hand or resting in the right axilla, it sometimes appeared in the left hand or left axilla. Some ancient writers attributed additional symbolism to the staff. Festus (third century AD), for example, described it as being gnarled in order to represent the difficulty of the physician's art (ET 691). Cornutus (first century AD) considered the staff symbolic of the support needed for health and to prevent recovery stumbling back to sickness (ET 705), while Eusebius (c300 AD) saw the staff as a symbol of support and relief for invalids (ET 706). This alternative function for the staff is corroborated by a marble statue in the Fitzwilliam Museum, Cambridge, England, which shows Asclepius carrying a long, crutch-like staff with a terminal cross bar for axillary support. Hippocrates mentioned a special significance for the staff:

> '...and the taking up of the staff happened to be celebrated on that day [annual 'Feast of the Asclepiads'], the annual festival, as you know, a solemn festival for us [people of Cos], and a magnificent procession to the cypress grove, which it was customary to be led by those who were related to the god'. Hippocrates in *Epistulae II* (ET 568)

This perhaps represented a ceremony equivalent to a present-day university convocation for awarding degrees to medical students.

The staff and serpent symbols used in medical coats of arms vary. For instance, the British Medical Association uses a stout staff (Figure 25), while the Canadian Medical Association's staff tapers to a point and is entwined by leaves symbolizing the ever-growing body of scientific knowledge used by the physician (Figure 26). The Royal College of Physicians and Surgeons of Canada uses a stout staff and a ferocious serpent (Figure 81).

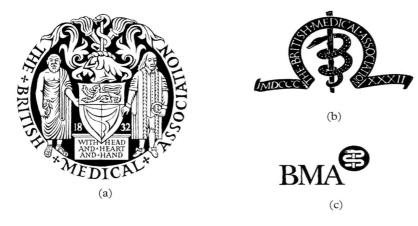

Figure 25 (a) The coat of arms of the British Medical Association. Its crest depicts a stout, straight staff entwined by a friendly serpent with a prominent forked tongue ready to give a 'healing lick'
(b) The 'Gill Logo' used for many years by the *British Medical Journal* and still used on the journal's 'press information' letterhead
(c) The current simplified logo of the British Medical Association with a straight staff and a serpent with a determined demeanour (all figures provided by the British Medical Association, London, England)

The combination of serpent and staff may have evolved from the natural tree-climbing abilities of *E. longissima,* making it easy for a domesticated snake to be taught to assume this posture. By such means, a pet serpent could be controlled in the same way that a pet dog or cat is constrained and directed by collar and lead.

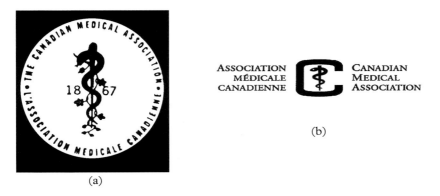

Figure 26 (a) Staff used by the Canadian Medical Association tapers almost to a needle-like point; it is entwined by a vine-like growth of maple leaves as well as by a serpent with protruding tongue (CMA)
(b) Simplified current logo of the Canadian Medical Association showing the tapering staff and a docile serpent (CMA)

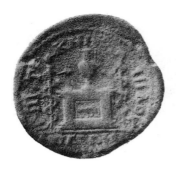

Figure 27   Coin of Pergamum showing altar with an ewer which is flanked by serpent-entwined, lighted torches (BMC, M&W)

Serpents of Asclepius were occasionally shown entwining altar lamps (Figure 27), and were also depicted encircling the omphalos of Delphi (Figure 12a).

Unusual depictions of serpents included the addition of wings and fiery breath, a version resulting in the creation of a dragon image. A coin from Pataulia depicts Asclepius, with his staff, riding on the back of a flying serpent. This symbolism may refer to Apollo[6]. A novel use of the serpent symbol occurred on the surgical forceps of the Coudee type, examples of which have been found both at Trier, Germany and at Littleborough, England[7]. The moulded tip of the forceps bears a serpent head used as a probe or elevator for lifting tendons, blood vessels and ligaments. The lower part, which would have been held by the surgeon, was shaped like a serpent's body. These instruments belonged to Roman surgeons who were Asclepiads. This ingenious design provided better manual control, as well as incorporating a talisman of Asclepius.

Fake serpents and false symbols

Alexander of Abonoteichus, known as the Fake Prophet, was born in the Black Sea territory of Paphlagonia in c105 AD. Much of our information on Alexander is derived from a hostile account by the second century Greek satirist, Lucian. Alexander is said to have begun his career as a boy prostitute and to have apprenticed himself to a notorious follower of the neopythagorean, Apollonius of Tyana in Asia Minor. Apollonius was a famed ascetic and wandering teacher, perhaps a pagan equivalent of Jesus Christ, although the details of his life remain uncertain. According to Lucian, Alexander's tutor was taught the 'whole bag of tricks' by Apollonius. He became a quack who, among other things, advertised love potions for those seeking to improve their sex life. Alexander learned his lessons well, with his tutor acting as both his teacher and lover.

At an early age, Alexander orchestrated a plan to reappear in his home city as the son of Podalirius. He arrived with a tame serpent named Glycon, which he concealed until he had convinced the townspeople into thinking they had discovered a baby serpent that was the reincarnation of Asclepius. He then constructed a model of a

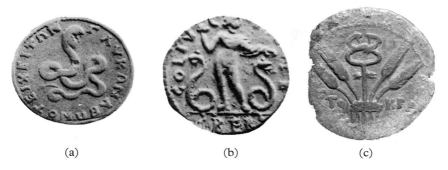

(a)   (b)   (c)

Figure 28
(a) Coin of Abonoteichus depicting Glycon (the False Serpent of Asclepius) (BMC, M&W)
(b) Coin of Berytus in Phoenicia showing Eshmun-Asclepius with twin serpents (GDH)
(c) Caduceus flanked by two ears of grain on a coin of Claudius from the Roman province of Egypt (41–54 AD). The caduceus symbolizes either Ceres or Commerce (GDH)

human head with long, curly hair and moving jaws, which he attached to the tail of his tame pet. The greatest medical and prophetic hoax of the second century AD was thus set as Alexander tucked the serpent under his arm and placed the tail, with its false head, through his beard[8]. He reviewed the written petitions that had been sent to him and used the artificial head as a ventriloquist's dummy to speak to people. Ordinary supplicants paid the equivalent of half a day's wages, but the wealthy, including senators and emperors, paid significantly higher amounts for his services. His 'act' became so famous that the human-headed serpent was depicted on the coins of Abonoteichus (Figure 28a), and a small, bronze sculpture was even discovered in Athens. These coins were used during the reigns of several emperors, from Antoninus Pius (138–61 AD) to Trebonianus Gallus (251–3 AD), and continued to be minted after Alexander's death in 171 AD, indicating that the false cult survived for another 80 years until Lucian revealed the chicanery. Lucian's story, 'Alexander the False Prophet', exposed Glycon and gave numismatists the earliest coin record of medical quackery[9].

Some medical writers have referred to the 'twin serpents of Asclepius' but these are not truly symbolic of him. There are a few isolated numismatic examples of these false symbols, one of which depicts the infant Asclepius while another, from Berytus in Phoenicia, shows Eshmun-Asclepius standing between two horned serpents (Figure 28b). Emperor Septimius Severus and his sons and heirs, Geta and Caracalla, minted a coin in the third century which depicted a nude god labelled by numismatists as 'Asclepius adolescens'. The god stood before a bistyle temple. In his right hand he held the symbolic serpent-entwined staff but is flanked on each side by two large, rearing serpents whose heads are turned upwards (Figure 10). These examples do not justify the term 'twin serpents' — in fact, the latter example probably depicted serpents associated with Apollo (see chapter 2).

The Greek astronomer Eudoxus of Cnidus (408–355 BC) noted that there was a constellation in Scorpion that showed a person with a serpent in both hands — this was called Ophiuchus (the Serpent-bearer). Scientists Eratosthenes (276–194 BC) and Hyginus, and the didactic poet Aratus (315 BC), later ascribed these stars to Asclepius who had been raised to the heavens as a favour to Apollo after being struck dead with a thunderbolt by Zeus (ET 121)[11].

Serpents were depicted on temple doors and on jambs beside the entrance. The two serpents on jambs were used to provide artistic symmetry rather than denoting Asclepius' twin serpents. The concept of the 'twin serpents' did not originate from these minor examples but was most likely the result of present-day physicians rationalizing their use of the caduceus — the symbol of Hermes (Mercury) (chapter 12) (Figure 28c). The caduceus also appeared on ancient coins with the following deities: Agathodaemon[12], Athena, Artemis, Demeter and her daughter, Core or Persephone, Apollo, the personifications of Good fortune Tyche (Greek), Felicity (Roman), the City of Rome (Roma). It also appears with a Gorgon and with Pax, who is shown guiding a serpent with a caduceus. In antiquity, the caduceus was never in fact used in association with Asclepius.

Notes and references

1. Gluckman LK. The staff of Asklepios. A theory of origin supported by clinical ethnopsychiatry. *N Z Med J* 1966; **65**: 111–8.
2. Arnold EN, Burton JA. *The field guide to the reptiles and amphibians of Britain and Europe*. London: Collins, 1978.
3. Laughlin VL. The Aesculapian staff and the caduceus as medical symbols. *J Int Col Surgeons* 1962; **37**(4): 82–92.
4. Schmidt KP, Inger RF. *Reptiles of the world*. New York: Hanover House, Garden City, 1957: 211. Schmidt and Inger state that a melanistic *Elaphe longissima* is a rare variant; this, however, contrasts to its ancient description given in *Scholia in Nicandrum, Ad Therica*, 438 (ET 698), which described the serpent as black.
5. Angeletti LR, Agrimi U, Curia C *et al*. Healing rituals and sacred serpents. *Lancet* 1992; **340**: 223–5.

6. Seeger P. The staff of Asclepios. *Image Roche* 1966; **14**: 29–32.
7. Jackson R, Leahy K. A Roman surgical forceps from near Littleborough and a note on type. *Britannia* 1990; **21**: 271–4.
8. Zorgniotti AW. Alexander of Abonoteichus: false priest of Asclepius. *JAMA* 1973; **224**: 87–9.
9. The depiction of quacks on coinage is not unique. English token coins of the 18th and 19th centuries advertised the extravagant cures of many quack remedies[10]. The most famous of these depicts the self-styled Professor Holloway on the obverse with Hygieia on the reverse. Holloway's claims were so extravagant that the depiction on the reverse should have been Panacea!
10. Hart GD. English token coins and medicine. *Can Med Assoc J* 1966; **95**: 1311–7.
11. Dr Jacqueline Mitton of the Royal Astronomical Society has confirmed the observations of Eudoxus of Cnidus and reported that there are 13 star signs in the zodiac and that all previous calculations are wrong. The sign Ophiuchus (Asclepius) occurs November 30 to December 17. (Reported in the *Daily Telegraph*, January 20 1995.)
12. Agathodaemon was the Greek god of good spirit, grain fields and vineyards. He was frequently depicted in works of art and on coins as a huge serpent. The *Encyclopaedia Britannica* states that the Greeks toasted him with a cup of pure wine at the end of each meal.

Chapter 4

Asclepian temples and religious practices

Temples

Asclepius was a terrestrial god, associated with specific places on the earth. He lived permanently in his temple (Asclepieion), in contrast with the Olympian gods who moved with agility from one place to another[1]. A prominent statue indicated his presence in the main temple building, and he was worshipped at an altar located within his sacred precinct. Temple facilities adapted to the increasing number of followers. A system of Asclepian temple medicine evolved that was practised at the ancient equivalent of a modern specialist medical centre. Most temples were situated in surroundings emphasizing the beauty of nature and the wonder of the gods, while others were built on prestigious sites such as the Acropolis of Athens and Rome's island in the Tiber. Knowledge of Asclepieia and their amenities has been obtained from classical literature, archaeology and numismatics.

Pollio Vitruvius, a Roman architect and engineer of the first century BC, designed these buildings with insight into the needs for successful healthcare. He realized the therapeutic effect of the temple on the healing process and was aware of potential pollution problems:

'Moreover it will be naturally fitting if, for all temples in the first place, the healthiest sites be chosen. Also suitable springs of water are necessary in those places where shrines are to be set up, and for Asclepius in particular and for Salus and for those gods by whose medical power a great many of the sick seem to be healed. For when the sick are moved from a disease-ridden to a healthy place and the water supply is from health-giving fountains, they will recover more quickly. So it will be the case that the godliness that derives from the nature of the site will lead to an even greater reputation and authority.' *De architectura*[2] volume 12, 7 (ET 707)

The main Asclepieia provided the following facilities: drinking water with special healing properties; water for bathing, ritual cleansing and hydrotherapy; gymnasia; theatre; *abaton* (dream room); exhibition and display of votives and testimonials; space for rituals, festivals and processions.

Temple waters

An adequate supply of water was essential for every temple and its source was usually a local spring. Asclepian temples demonstrated ingenuity in their use of engineering hydraulics using channels, cisterns, reservoirs, aqueducts and fountains to supply the various amenities.

In addition to water being necessary for life and hygiene, it was an essential component of ritual and therapy. Water symbolized continuity with the depths of the earth and communication with the chthonian deities. A hot spring promoted the therapeutic and theurgical properties of the water.

The Temple of Sulis Minerva in Bath, England, was the most notable of Roman Britain — 250,000 gallons of water, at 46.5 °C, continues to flow daily from the chthonian depths of the earth even today. The copious supply of water catered for the popular pastime of the bath ritual. This ritual provided comfort, relaxation and an opportunity for social discourse. Supplicants were invigorated, experienced improved muscle tone, and found various aches and pains due to arthritis, rheumatism and fibrositis to be relieved. Warm baths were considered beneficial to the assimilation of food, reflecting an observation of the post-prandial need for increased blood circulation to the gastrointestinal tract. If a natural hot spring was not available, water was heated for bathing. The bathing ritual included baths with graduated changes in temperature. Today's sauna incorporates the extremes of the ritual including the cold plunge into a frigid pool.

Pilgrims were required to purify themselves with water from the sacred fountain. The temple ritual included bathing for cleanliness and repeated use of the various bath house amenities in order to create inner relaxation and ablution of accumulated stresses. Regular imbibing of temple water, with its medicinal and psychological properties, increased the daily intake of fluids.

Vitruvius also described the effects of local geology on the taste of water and its additives. Hot springs were enhanced by the presence of alum, bitumen or sulphur in the sub-surfaces of the earth; this influenced the taste, therapeutic properties and alkalinity or acidity of the water. Experience led Vitruvius to state that sulphur springs refreshed muscular weakness by 'heating and burning off poisonous humours from the body'[2] — today, we would feel that the heat increased circulation, especially to inflamed areas, and the resulting capillary dilatation removed local inflammatory metabolites. Vitruvius thought alum was beneficial to body parts dissolved by paralysis or disuse (his dissolution of paralysis was the atrophy (wasting) of muscles resulting from the interruption of its motor nerve supply). Muscles affected as such are treated today by hydrotherapy (in chlorinated water), where buoyancy of the limb helps movement and tone of a paralysed muscle. Bitumen furnished 'draughts which purge and heal inner defects' but bathing waters containing bitumen (tar) treated a variety of skin ailments, especially psoriasis where 'the inner defect' is an excess multiplication of the cells in the basal (interior) layer of the skin. Imbibing alkaline water purged the intestines and drinking acid spring water dissolved bladder stones. Vitruvius even recorded that some of the water in the Alps caused goitre — this region continues to be an endemic goitre area today[2,3]. Hot and cold baths, or hot and cold drinks, were used to correct excesses of warm or cold humours and the fluids per se were used to remedy excess dry humours (see chapter 8).

The three most famous Asclepian temples were located at Epidaurus, Cos and Pergamum. Their extensive facilities earned them an international reputation which attracted the rich and famous, as well as those with severe illnesses.

Asclepieion of Epidaurus — the Holy City (ET 400)
The earliest and most illustrious Asclepieion was founded at Epidaurus in the sixth century BC. Viewed by a physician, this temple design is better suited to patient care than that at Cos or Pergamum due to its inclusion of ramps which provided user-friendly access to individuals suffering from arthritis, heart and respiratory disease and debilitation. The immensity of the ancient complex is described in Papadakis' modern guidebook to Epidaurus[4], which lists the following features: propylaea (monumental gateway); sacred way and sacred place; hexastyle temple of Asclepius; tholos (a rotunda with 26 Doric columns); *abaton* or *encoimeterion* (sleeping area); 70-metre-long colonnade; great altar of Asclepius; possible ancient *abaton*; hexastyle temple of Artemis; palaestra (exercise room); stoa of Cotys; propylaea of the gymnasium; gymnasium; Roman odeum (roofed theatre); Greek baths; guest house; temple of the Egyptian Apollo and Asclepius; Roman baths; north portico (porch); temple of Aphrodite; baths of Asclepius; library; temple of Themis (goddess of order and justice); and stadium and theatre. The complex also included a sacred fountain and votive tablets describing cures of actual patients[4] (Plan 1).

Plan 1   Asclepieion of Epidaurus

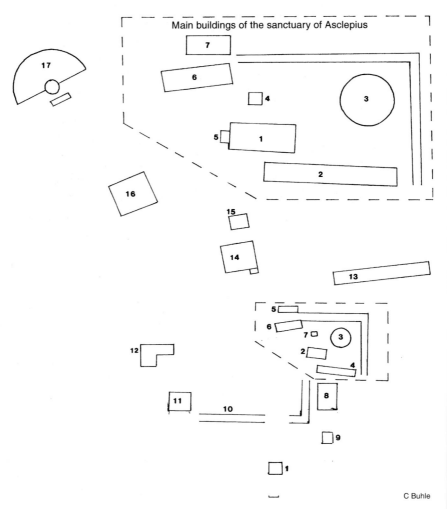

C Buhle

1. Propylea
2. Temple of Asclepius
3. Tholos
4. *Abaton*
5. Temple of Artemis
6. Ancient *abaton*
7. Great altar
8. Library
9. Temple of Aphrodite
10. Portico
11. Roman baths
12. Temple of Egyptian Apollo and Asclepius
13. Stadium
14. Gymnasium
15. Greek baths
16. Guest house
17. Theatre

Main buildings of the sanctuary of Asclepius

1. Temple of Asclepius
2. *Abaton*
3. Tholos
4. Great altar
5. Sacred fountain
6. Ancient *abaton*
7. Temple of Artemis

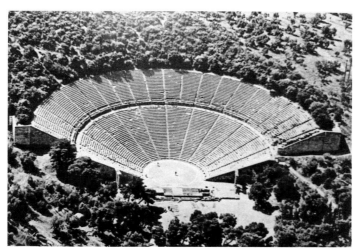

Figure 29   Theatre at Epidaurus (Photo © Office National du Tourisme Grec, Montreal, Quebec, Canada)

The recovered architectural fragments, displayed in the Museum of Epidaurus, express the epitome of classical aesthetic excellence. The facades of the buildings, decorated with intricate designs and floral patterns, created a panorama of harmony in marble. Pausanias, a travel writer of the second century AD, described Epidaurus in *Descriptio Graecae II*, 27 (ET 739) providing a contemporary comment on the surviving archaeological remains. His detailed description of individual buildings is beyond the scope of this book but a brief summary is outlined below, starting with the theatre, to emphasize the magnitude of facilities dedicated to an holistic approach to healthcare.

'In the sanctuary of Epidaurus there is a theatre that, in my opinion, is really well worth seeing . . . when it comes to symmetry and beauty, what architect could vie with Polyclitus? For it was Polyclitus, who made the theatre and the circular building also.' (Pausanias ET 739)

Polyclitus lived and worked in the mid-fourth century BC. The theatre survived the centuries and was reopened in 1954 with a revival of the Epidauria — the annual Athenian festival of Asclepius. The perfect acoustics achieved in antiquity allow a present-day audience of 14,000 spectators to hear the actors without using an electronic sound system! This is lasting architectural testimony to the ancient Greek philosophers who sought harmony with the forces of nature for attainment of the ideal (Figure 29).

The circular building referred to by Pausanias was the tholos, built between 370 and 330 BC. One of the most beautiful buildings of ancient Greece, its exterior design was a symphonic composition of marble and sculpture, with an interior richly decorated by the paintings of Pausias:

> '... Eros who has thrown away his bow and arrows, and has picked up a lyre instead. Here is also another painting, which is also by Pausias: Drunkenness is drinking out of a goblet made of crystal; and in the picture you can see the crystal goblet and through it the face of a woman.' (Pausanias, ET 739)

The original purpose of the tholos remains unknown but historians have suggested its use for banquets, religious ceremonies, literary contests, and even as the temple treasury. Its mysterious underground labyrinth has been suggested as the site of the snake-pit and home of the Epidaurian serpents thought to be the embodiment of Asclepius (Ovid *Metamorphoses XV*, 622–744; ET 850, chapter 8). This theory is supported by Kerenyi's description of the discovery of a rodent stone carving[5] at that site, and by the presence of underground, circular pits similar to those found at sites associated with Apollo[6]. Papadakis states that the labyrinth of the tholos was probably the burial place of the hero-god Asclepius and his 'heroic' and chthonian nature secretly honoured in this subterranean site while the divine Asclepius was worshipped publicly above ground at the temple.

The main temple was built between 380 and 375 BC by the architect Theodotos and richly decorated by Thrasymedes and Timotheos, who were among the foremost artists of that era. The cult statue of Asclepius, described by Pausanias, was its most outstanding feature:

> 'Asclepius' statue is half the size of the statue of Olympian Zeus at Athens: it is made of ivory and gold. An inscription informs us that the sculptor was Thrasymedes from Paros. The god is seated on a throne clutching a staff, whilst holding his other hand over the head of a serpent; and a dog, lying beside him, is also represented. On the throne there are carved in relief the deeds of the Argive heroes: Bellerophon fighting the Chimaera and Perseus who is carrying off Medusa's head.'[7] (ET 739)

Thrasymedes sculpted the statue around 375 BC. This work of art miraculously escaped destruction by Sulla in 86 BC when he sacked all the sanctuaries of Greece to pay for his war against Mithridates. Sulla probably remembered Asclepius' saving of Rome in 292 BC and feared reprisal. Nothing of the statue remains today but, fortunately, a contemporary coin of Epidaurus records this famous depiction of Asclepius (Figure 6a). A fourth century BC coin and a second century AD coin of Epidaurus depicted the Thrasymedes statue located in a tetrastyle temple.

Pausanias also described: 'Inside the grove is a temple of Artemis and an image of Epione; also a sanctuary of Aphrodite and Themis; and a stadium formed, like most Greek stadia, by mounds of raised earth; there is also a fountain worth seeing for its roof and for its general magnificence'. (ET 739)

Testimonies of cure were an important part of Asclepian temple medicine. Pausanias recorded: 'Six votive tablets inscribed with the names of men and women who were healed by Asclepius, together with the disease from which each suffered, and the way in which each was cured'. (ET 739)

Two of these marble stelae, inscribed by temple priests in the sixth to fourth century BC, were found in the *abaton* and are exhibited in the museum[4]. Most of these cures are examples of the priest's ability to cure by the power of mind over body, with the exception of one recording: 'A dog cured a boy from Aegina who had a growth on his neck. When he came into the presence of the God, one of the sacred dogs healed him using its tongue while he was awake and cured him.' (ET 423)

Could the growth have been an abscess or a cyst ruptured by the massaging pressure of the dog's lick? The depiction of a dog lying beside Asclepius in the statue by Thrasymedes alludes to the Epidaurian belief that a dog guarded the child Asclepius. A dog's lick was thought to have healing properties, especially for eye diseases — dogs played a role in some of the healing shrines of Asclepius and at a few Celtic shrines. The reverse of another Asclepian coin from Epidaurus depicts one of the temple dogs (Figure 30). This resembles the Irish wolfhound-like hunting dog found at the temple of Nodens at Lydney[8].

The temple's guest house was a large structure built like an American motel. It comprised 160 rooms that were contained in four

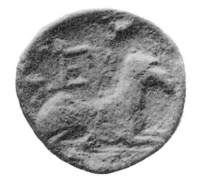

Figure 30 Coin (323–240 BC) depicting Asclepius' sacred dog from Epidaurus. Its size suggests descent from the hunting dogs of Apollo Maleatus and it would certainly be capable of a large, therapeutic lick. The obverse depicts Asclepius (BMC, M&W)

76-metre-long blocks surrounding a central courtyard. The modern, cost-effective concept of housing patients in hotels or motels rather than hospitals is perhaps not so modern after all!

The *abaton* was the sacred place where patients slept and were cured by Asclepius. This was a colonnaded structure 70 metres in length using the slope of the ground, which became a split-level building. In the second century AD, Pausanias recorded the extensive Roman renovations at Epidaurus:

> 'The buildings put up in our own day by the Roman Senator Antoninus include a bath of Asclepius; ... a temple to Hygieia, as well as to Asclepius and Apollo...and a *stoa* (portico) called the Stoa of Cotys.' (ET 739)

The temple to Health (Hygieia or Salus) was built in the propylaea of the original gymnasium. Pausanias describes the custom, at Epidaurus and other Asclepian temples, of excluding from the area dying patients and women about to give birth:

> 'The sacred grove of Asclepius is surrounded by boundaries on every side. No one should be allowed to die and no woman be allowed to give birth within the enclosure; just the same practice is observed in the Island of Delos.' (ET 739)

These are surprising regulations for temples of the god of medicine. The policy of excluding the dying may be ascribed to the Asclepian myth in which Zeus prohibited Asclepius from reviving the dead, although it is more likely to have had pragmatic origins. Their exclusion reduced the spread of fatal infectious diseases. The presence of dying patients, along with their grief-stricken relatives, would reduce the ambience of the temple's healing environment. The priests understood the anger grieving relatives sometimes felt against those caring for their loved ones, but they were also aware of the fact that expressing these emotions would adversely effect the reputation and mystique of the Asclepieion and its healing potential. Women patients ready to give birth were probably excluded on the basis of the vocalization accompanying parturition in Mediterranean countries. In those days, as today, babies seemed to come at night, thus their delivery would have disturbed the ritual healing temple sleep of supplicants. Pausanias records the sensitivity of the Epidaurians towards these people:

'The Epidaurians around the sanctuary were in great distress, because the women folk were not allowed to give birth under shelter and their sick were obliged to die under the open sky. In order to remedy this state of affairs, Antoninus established a building in which people may die [echoes of the hospice movement and the forerunner of today's palliative care units] and a woman may give birth to her baby [today's delivery room suite] without causing offence to the God.' (ET 488)

The formal gateway (propylaea) to the sacred temple at Epidaurus was a classical arch with six marble Ionian columns on both the inside and outside. Above the arch appeared a rhyming inscription expounding the philosophical basis of Asclepian worship. It is surprising that Pausanias did not record this inscription but perhaps his omission reflects an interest biased towards architecture rather than philosophical matters. Fortunately, several ancient writers recorded the words: 'Anyone who enters this temple, fragrant with incense, must be pure; purity means to think nothing but holy thoughts'. Porphyrius, *De Abstinentia*, II, 19 (ET 318) This inscription was a guide for supplicants seeking help — holy thoughts gave the necessary harmony needed to heal body and soul.

The temple of Epidaurus, and probably most Asclepian temples, was fragranced by burning incense. This ritual went beyond pleasing Asclepius — it also dispelled odours and contagion carried by those who would not have received full marks for cleansing before entering the temple. Perhaps there was also an ancient added dash of aromatherapy! A coin of Epidaurus, minted between 323 BC and

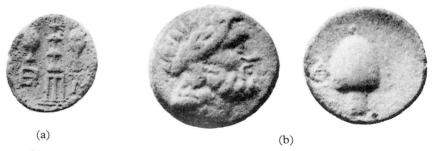

(a)   (b)

Figure 31
(a) The reverse of a coin of Epidaurus (323–240 BC) showing an altar on which two cupping vessels flank a *thymiaterion*. The obverse of this coin type depicts either Asclepius or Apollo and symbolizes that, at that time, Apollo had not completely retired from practice (Photo BMC, M&W)
(b) The obverse of a coin from Epidaurus depicting Asclepius and on the reverse a large cupping vessel (323–240 BC) (Photo BMC, M&W)

240 BC, depicted two cupping vessels flanking a *thymiaterion* or censer used for burning incense (Figure 31a). The coins in Figure 31 have great historical significance because cupping vessels associated with the temple demonstrate the combination of medical practice with theurgical ritual at the Asclepieia (see chapter 8).

The Goths destroyed Epidaurus in 395 AD. Its brief revival terminated in 426 AD when Emperor Theodosius II ordered its gates closed. Two great earthquakes during the sixth century AD affected its total and final destruction.

Asclepieion of Cos — the Sacred Island (ET 7)

The Asclepieion of Cos was situated on top of a hill surrounded by pines, giving approaching supplicants an inspiring view of the majestic temple site. Unfortunately, this formidable location needed many steps making access difficult for weak and handicapped patients. Hippocrates established a medical school at Cos in the fifth century BC. His fame as a physician did much to establish Cos as the 'Sacred Island' of Asclepius. He is thought to have taught under a plane tree, reputed to be the oldest tree in Europe[9,10]. The following description of the temple at Cos may be gleaned from the poetic writings of the third century BC Herondas (*Mimiambi* IV, 195) (ET 482):

> In the forecourt of the temple there was an altar on which sacrifices were burnt. On each side, there were statues executed by the sons of Praxiteles; these depicted the family of Asclepius (Apollo, Coronis, Epione, Hygieia, Panacea, Iaso, Podalirius, and Machaon). There were other statues with fine artistic merit and appeal, as well as votives and gifts. Located in the *cella* of the temple was the cult statue of the god and the temple instruments. The walls were decorated with images of such realism that a woman visitor had to stifle a scream because an oxen was viewing her with a threatening eye.

Modern archaeological excavations have revealed a temple complex on three separate terraces linked by stairways (Figure 32) (Plan 2)[10]. The lower terrace, approached by a stairway of 24 steps, contained patient facilities including rooms, a heated bath, mineral springs and the medical school. It features an inscription to the Coan physician Xenophon, famed for the political favours he gained from Emperor Claudius. The second terrace, 30 steps above the first, contained the high altar to Asclepius and temples to Asclepius and Apollo. The uppermost terrace, reached by a further 60 steps, housed the second

Plan 2   Asclepieion of Cos

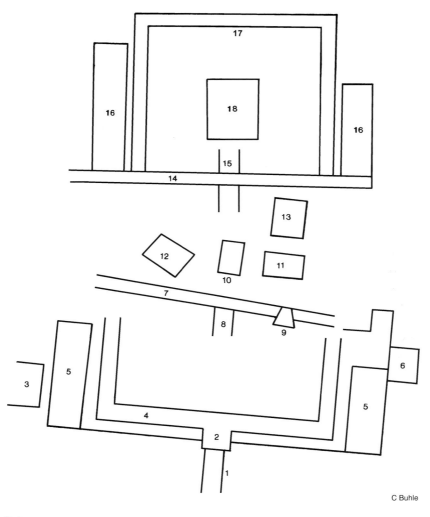

C Buhle

1. Stairway
2. Propylaea
3. Thermae
4. Portico
5. Rooms for patients
6. Latrines
7. Terraced wall
8. Stairway
9. Temple to Xenophon

10. Altar of Asclepius
11. Ionic temple of Asclepius
12. Corinthian temple of Asclepius
13. Rooms for priests
14. Terraced wall
15. Stairway
16. Rooms for patients
17. Portico
18. Temple of Asclepius

century BC Doric-style temple of Asclepius which measured 34 metres by 18 metres and featured 104 columns. This level also housed large statues of Asclepius and Hygieia. At its eastern end stood a column with a Christian inscription and a surmounting marble slab. There is

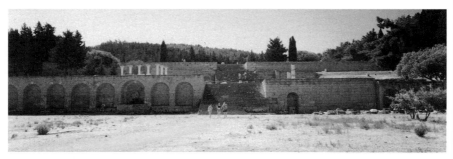

Figure 32 Modern view of the Asclepieion at Cos (Photo by Mrs Jill Robertson, Toronto, ON, Canada)

no evidence of ramps for wheelchair access—perhaps patients with arthritic and other disabilities were first cured at the medical school clinics on the first level, and then were able to climb the 114 steps to thank Asclepius. The steps indicate the preference of the priests for protocol and grandeur, and emphasize their control of access to Asclepius. This probably maintained their prestige and position over and above Hippocrates and other physicians associated with the island.

The coinage of Cos did not reflect the prominence of Asclepius on the island until about 166–88 BC, but Coan coinage of the second century AD shows the earliest depictions of actual physicians, with portraits of a balding Hippocrates and of Xenophon (Figures 20a & 58). Despite the rise of Christianity and the fall of paganism, the Asclepieion of Cos continued to function until 554 AD when it was destroyed by an earthquake. It is difficult to date the Christian inscriptions but their presence conforms to the Christian practice of adopting and adapting pagan sites (chapter 11).

Asclepieion of Pergamum — the hearth of Asclepius (ET 402)
The Asclepieion at Pergamum was founded in about 350 BC by Archias, who supplied the necessary temple serpents from Epidaurus after his recovery there from a hunting injury (ET 709 & 801). Pergamum became the largest Asclepian sanctuary in Asia Minor, its importance demonstrated by the extensive archaeological remains and emphasized by the many coins that preserve a unique record of its architectural features. In 133 BC, it became the capital of the Roman province of Asia and, hence, the most important Roman city in the area known today as the Middle East.

Several coins portraying the architectural masterpieces of the ancient world are reviewed in Donaldson's book, *Architectura numismatica*[11]. Many buildings of antiquity, now vanished without trace, have had their form preserved on a contemporary coin. The most prominent of

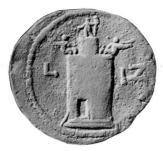

Figure 33   Coin of Alexandria (117–38 AD) depicting the Pharos of Alexandria. The structure was completely destroyed by an earthquake and ancient coins are the only record of its form. Some coins depict it as a square tower while others depict a circular tower (Photo Cast from British Museum (BMC), M&W)

these is the Pharos of Alexandria (Figure 33). The accuracy of ancient numismatic portraiture is demonstrated by a coin depicting Emperor Titus commemorating the opening of the Colosseum in 80 AD. This medallion shows an aerial view of the Colosseum displaying the architectural detail seen today. It also portrays the rows of statues that once lined the upper galleries and the enormous columnar fountain, the Meta Sudans, which originally stood alongside the structure.

Coins of Cos do not show the architecture of its temple, while those of Epidaurus show that the Thrasymedes statue was located in a tetrastyle temple. Coins of Pergamum depict different architecture from the wellknown reconstruction by Shleif (Figure 34)[12], and their

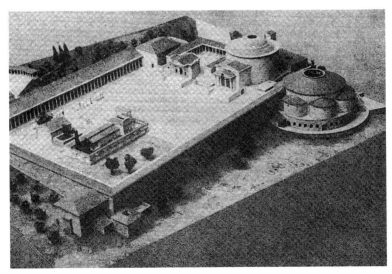

Figure 34   Artistic reconstruction of Pergamum in the middle of the third century AD before the earthquake, based on archaeological evidence (Photo from Image reproduced with the permission of Hoffman-La Roche Ltd, Mississauga, ON, Canada)

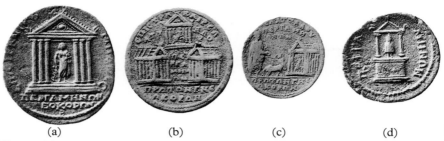

(a)   (b)   (c)   (d)

Figure 35
(a) Coin of Commodus (180–92 AD) from Pergamum showing a hexastyle temple with Asclepius standing and holding a serpent-entwined staff (Photo BMC, M&W)
(b) Coin of Caracalla (214 AD) from Pergamum depicting two pentastyle temples flanking a tetrastyle with a seated Asclepius holding a serpent-entwined staff (Photo BMC, M&W)
(c) Coin of Pergamum (214 AD) showing Asclepius in a tetrastyle temple. In the forecourt, Caracalla and humped bull about to be struck a blow by youth beyond (Photo BMC, M&W)
(d) Coin of Commodus (180–92 AD) showing Telesphorus in his own bistyle temple (Photo BMC, M&W)
Coins b & c commemorated Caracalla's visit to Pergamum in 214 AD; they were probably minted in order to gain favour or give thanks to Asclepius for successful treatment

coin date may indicate that the tholos was built after Caracalla's visit in 214 AD. Temples of many other gods were portrayed on coins of Pergamum but the temple of Asclepius predominated. These depictions served as an ancient counterpart for travel posters or postcards, allowing people in distant places to visualize the greatness of the 'hearth' of Asclepius at Pergamum. The coins could also serve as talismans for those cured of disease.

Coins depict Pergamum's Asclepian temple complex as a series of buildings, the main temple being hexastyle with a pedimented front supported on six Doric columns. At the centre was an immense cult statue of Asclepius, standing with his serpent-entwined staff held in his right hand. Two pentastyle temples (five columns) flanked a quadrastyle temple (four columns) housing a statue of Asclepius seated on his throne. There was a sacrificial forecourt in front of the quadrastyle temple and a bistyle temple (two columns) dedicated to Telesphorus, as well as additional prominent statues of Asclepius (Figures 35a & b). These coins do not illustrate the two circular buildings whose foundations remain, suggesting these structures were built after the dates of the coins (Plan 3). The classical style of the buildings portrayed on coins differs from the Schlief reconstruction emphasizing two circular buildings. Were the circular buildings built after 214 AD? If this was not the case then this is an example of an

Plan 3   Asclepieion of Pergamum

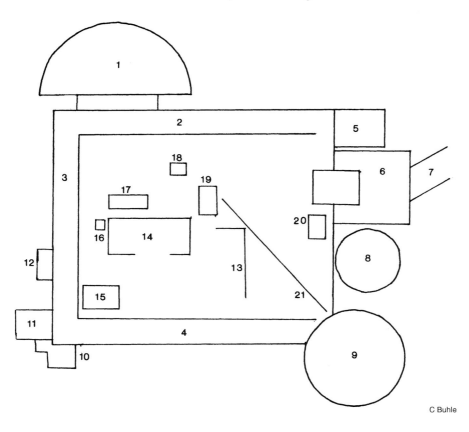

C Buhle

1. Theatre
2. North gallery
3. West gallery
4. South gallery
5. Library
6. Propylaea
7. Holy Road
8. Temple of Zeus-Asclepius
9. Tholos
10. Lavatories
11. Large west room

12. Small west room
13. Hellenistic wall
14. Incubation room
15. Roman temples
16. Well
17. Temple of Asclepius Soter
18. Altar
19. Holy springs
20. Cult niche
21. Subterranean passage

inaccurate numismatic record because the archaeology attests to the presence of the circular buildings.

The massive size of the Asclepian cult statues is emphasized by the coins in Figures 35a & b. The depiction of the temple key on a coin indicates temple security and the need to prevent nocturnal supplicants from disturbing those undergoing the incubation ritual (Figure 36a). The director of the gymnasium was sufficiently important to be depicted on coins. In 31 BC, Pergamum depicted a basin on a coin

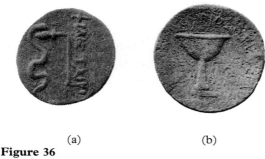

(a)   (b)

Figure 36
(a) Coin from Pergamum (211–130 BC) depicting a
temple key with a serpent on the reverse (the obverse
shows Asclepius) (Photo BMC, M&W)
(b) Coin from Pergamum (27 BC–14 AD) showing
a basin probably associated with hydrotherapy and
inscribed '*gymnasiarch*' (master of the gymnasium)
(Photo BMC, M&W)

bearing the inscription '*gymnasiarch*' (master of the gymnasium) (Figure 36b) and in 98 AD Anazarbos issued a coin depicting a man standing before a basin, also inscribed '*gymnasiarch.*' A large ancillary staff was necessary to supply, maintain and clean the temple complex, theatre, stadium and gymnasium, guesthouse or hotel and all the other facilities. Coins of the first century BC from here were the first to proclaim that Asclepius was the saviour, with the Greek inscription 'soter' accompanying his portrait on the obverse. The reverse displays either the staff and serpent symbol or a snake-entwined omphalos. Other coins of Pergamum depict a variety of other gods — one issue even combines Athena on the obverse with the staff and serpent symbol on the reverse.

Emperor Caracalla's visit to Pergamum in 214 AD was commemorated on several coins. He was depicted entering the city, sacrificing to Asclepius and paying homage to Asclepius, Telesphorus and the sacred serpent (Figure 21). Caracalla had several physical and psychological problems and sought help from many healing deities in the empire. He minted coins elsewhere depicting Asclepius; in fact a general circulation silver denarius with a good portrait of the emperor on the obverse and Asclepius with or without Telesphorus on the reverse is one of the most readily available Asclepian coins. These may have been minted as a follow-up from vows made at Pergamum, or as an ongoing plea for help.

A heavily eroded stone found by archaeologists at Pergamum has provided one of the only surviving descriptions of the role of purification in the incubation ritual. Hakka Gultekin, of the Archaeological Museum of Izmir, Turkey, translated the inscription:

'The sick man shall go . . . ten days pass . . . he shall wash himself . . . take off his every day clothes and put on a white *chiton* . . . he shall gird himself with clean towels . . . approach God . . . he who seeks healing shall go into the large bedchamber . . . white sacrificial lambs

adorned with holy olive branches... wear neither ring nor girdle...
and walk barefoot.'[12]

Aelius Aristides, a man of letters in the second century AD, in *Oratio*
XXXIX, 118 (ET 409) in referring to the god Asclepius, describes the
spring in the centre of the temple complex at Pergamum:

'... this [spring] was discovered by and belongs to the great miracle-
worker [Asclepius], he who does everything for the healthy wellbeing
of humankind and for many it takes the place of drugs. For many
who have bathed in it recovered their eyesight, while many by
drinking were cured of chest ailments and regained vital breathing.
For in some cases it cured their feet, while for others it cured some
other part of the body. One patient who had been mute drank it and
straight away recovered his voice, just as those who drink sacred
waters turn into prophets. For some patients the process of drawing
off the water was itself therapeutic. What is more, it not only
provides a remedy and salvation for the sick, but even to those who
are enjoying good health, it renders the use of any other water
inappropriate.'

This quotation illustrates one of the essentials of temple medicine,
namely the physical or psychological curing powers of the temple
spring. The Pergamum spring should have been dedicated to Panacea
or cure-all! The use of the curative power of spring water continues to
this day and the testimonial of Aristides reads like an 18th to 20th
century advertisement for the waters of various European and North
American health spas.

Pergamum acquired a library which was exceeded only by Alexandria
in size and fame. Unfortunately, all was lost when an earthquake
destroyed Pergamum c253–60 AD. The temple was never rebuilt and
its site was robbed and quarried until the Christians paid Asclepius the
ultimate insult by using the site as a consecrated cemetery.

Smaller Asclepieia and the temple of Nodens
The ground plan of the average Asclepieion is similar to sanctuaries
dedicated to other divinities, the difference being that Asclepieia
included an *abaton*[13] and provided accommodation facilities for
supplicants. The average or smaller provincial Asclepian temple had a
basic plan similar to the one used at the Asclepian-style temple of
Nodens at Lydney, Gloucestershire, England, where a temple was
built in the post-Roman late fourth century AD on the site of an Iron-
Age hillfort and disused iron mines. Vitruvius could not have chosen a

Plan 4   Temple of Lydney

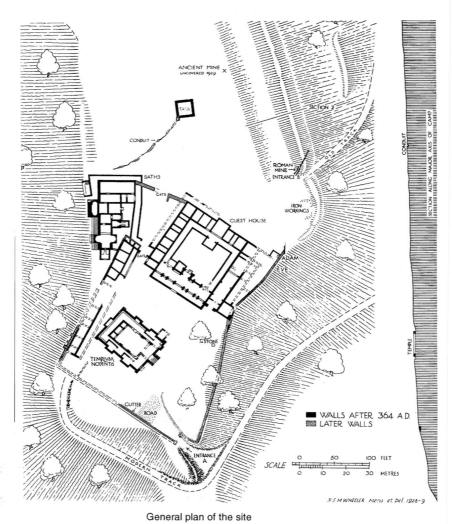

General plan of the site

The Society of Antiquaries of London

more beautiful and healthy location. The plan of this temple, formulated after its excavation by Wheeler and Wheeler in 1928–9, is shown in Plan 4[14]. Its nave, aisle, piscina and chapels are laid out in a basilican plan, unique for Britain at that time. Behind the temple stood a long building or *abaton* with a range of small rooms opening onto a veranda which, according to the excavators, resembled the *abata* at Epidaurus, Cos and Athens. This structure may have been used as shops selling and affixing votives in the temple, but its mosaic flooring makes this prosaic usage unlikely. Nodens had a large bathhouse and a guesthouse with an entrance hall, as well as a central paved courtyard surrounded by a veranda with rooms leading from it. This was not unlike the hotel at Epidaurus. A large stone basin projecting from the wall of the guesthouse may have been used for taking therapeutic water.

Healing votives were found at this site — one of these still held the pin fastening it to the wall. The finding of an oculist's stamp, inscribed with precise clinical instructions, is evidence for the availability of ancillary medical healing. Variations of this Lydney plan exist at many Asclepian temple sites.

Religious or cult practices

Alice Walton's book, *The cult of Asklepios*[15], describes the worship and rituals associated with Asclepius — the word 'cult' is also used by the Edelsteins to describe these activities. Although the term applies to all followers of ancient gods, it is inappropriate to associate it with Asclepius in the 20th century because a 'medical cult' practises unscientific quackery based on false or non-existent theories. Followers of Asclepius received medical care of the highest professional standard and were not members of what is today described as a medical cult.

The priests of the 'saviour Asclepius' had the highest authority at the Asclepieion, directing sacrifices and maintaining the regulations of worship. The rituals of supplicants had to be followed faithfully in order to obtain a cure. Priests administered 'mind-therapy' to selected patients and decided the duration of preliminary preparation for the final stage of the temple ritual, which was cure by incubation in the *abaton*. They were also responsible for recording gifts and auditing temple finances, a role similar to that of modern day hospital administrators. A hierarchy of subordinates assisted the priest in the various religious duties and ceremonies, and included the following: *neocorus* (*nacoros* in the local dialect) or sacred officer or assistant priest of some distinction; *pyrophoros* or the priest's assistant who 'bears the fire'; *zacoros* or attendant assisting the *neocoros*; *naophylakes* or temple guardians; *hieromnemones* who remembered the sacred words; and *aoidoi* or cantors[4].

The Edelsteins state that the priesthood did not need special training or experience. This conclusion may have been true for the later years of

Asclepian temple medicine, when temple cures were accompanied by medical treatment, but in archaic times the priests cured supplicants with mind therapy requiring both skill and experience.

Entry into the priesthood can accurately be described as nepotistic because choice was restricted to certain families who were known for their high spirituality and who jealously guarded the sacred traditions and secret rites. Most priests were elected to their position after gaining experience in one or more of the lower echelons of the temple hierarchy. The term of office was usually for one year but re-election for a second term was possible. The priesthood was hereditary at Pergamum, Mytilene and Lebena. Socrates (470–399 BC), friend and teacher of Plato, was one of the most influential philosophers of antiquity. He believed in Asclepius and served one term as priest at the Asclepieion of Athens.

Temples held daily morning and evening services at which most supplicants were healthy followers who prayed for continued health and the prevention of disease (Ritual for the health, Edelstein *II Interpretation*: 182–4). 'The gods are naturally well-disposed to do you good, but when invoked they are even better'. Libianus, *Declamations*, XXXIV, 23–6 (ET 538)

Some areas of the temple compound were accessible at night; here supplicants slept in the hope of receiving divine favour. Relatives and friends often prayed for patients at temple services and some even became surrogate patients during the incubation ritual. Prayer rather than sacrifice was the main component of daily liturgy and full-time choirs along with the congregation sang hymns:

'Wake up, Paeon Asclepius, lord of humanity, gentle-minded child of Leto's son and of noble Coronis, disperse sleep from your eyes and listen to the prayers of those who call upon you. We, your worshippers, rejoicing greatly, propitiate your prime power, Health, gentle-minded Asclepius; awake and be pleased to listen to your hymn, you whom we call upon with cries of "Hail!"' *Epigrammata Graeca*, 1027 (ET 598)

'... and the loud cry both of those who are present and of those who are arriving, shouting this very well-known refrain, "Great is Asclepius".' Aristides, *Oratio* XLVIII, 21 (ET 602)

The choirs and cantors may have been an early form of music therapy, creating an environmental ambience and contributing to inner calm and optimism among the congregation.

At inauspicious times the state would attempt to propitiate Asclepius to ward off a public disaster such as plague, famine or flood. Livy recorded a '*Salus Publica*' ceremony of great magnitude:

'The decemvirs proclaimed two days of prayer for health, not only in the city but in all the rural settlements and communities; all people over the age of twelve, wearing crowns and carrying laurel branches in their hands, made the supplication.' *Ab Urbe Condita*, XL, 37, 2–3 (ET 505)

The incubation ritual, central and unique to the success of the Asclepieia, is described in chapter 5. In addition, sacrifices formed part of all ancient religious practices and at Asclepieia, the custom was practised outside the principal temple using small animals such as rams or cocks. Goat sacrifice was forbidden in Epidaurus but permitted in Athens and other locations outside Thessaly. On major ceremonial occasions, especially when a prominent political figure was present, a bull and several animals were offered. Parts of the sacrifice were often given to the priest but this was not the custom at Epidaurus. The dying words of Socrates (399 BC) were: 'Crito, we owe a cock to Asclepius. Pay it and do not neglect it, do so!' Plato, *Phaedo* (ET 524). This resulted in the cock becoming symbolic of Asclepius. The sacrifice of this bird, noted for its watchfulness and morning crowing which scared away the spirits of darkness, was believed to prevent illness and ease childbirth. It continues to be sacrificed in Greece today as a good luck talisman when the foundations of a new house are being laid. The cock was also sacred to Apollo, Hermes, Ares, Core and Helius.

Entertainment was an integral part of any sojourn in a major Asclepian sanctuary such as Epidaurus or Pergamum, where the facilities included a small covered odeum, large amphitheatre, stadium, library, baths and other amenities including gambling tables. The odeum was used for performances before small audiences. Here, new authors were given an opportunity to read their prose or recite their poems. Entertainment was sometimes provided by patients who had been instructed to compose poems or prose while awaiting the incubation ceremony. This activity is comparable to present-day occupational therapy designed to stimulate interest and relieve depression and introspection. The Greeks knew the therapeutic benefit of laughter and even the gods were not immune from their barbs. Aristophanes (c446–385 BC) poked fun at Asclepius in his play, *Plutus*, when he recorded the experience of Carion, an observer present at an incubation ceremony:

Carion: And then I did something that will make you laugh; for as he [Asclepius] came near me, I let out a fart. I couldn't hold it in.
His wife: I bet the god was disgusted.
Carion: No, but it brought blushes to Iaso's cheeks and Panacea turned away her head and held her nose: my wind's no frankincense!
His wife: But what did he do?
Witness: Nothing, by Zeus, he wasn't bothered. (ET 421)[16]

The Greeks had also discovered the therapeutic benefit of a catharsis of emotions accompanying the performance of a tragedy. For instance, in Euripides' *Medea*, the heroine murders her two young children to spite her estranged husband, Jason, with whom she had originally eloped to Greece from her native country by the Black Sea. After such intense emotional experiences, patients perceived the personal problems in their lives as trifling and their psyches became tranquillized. As a result of these rituals, some of the finest theatres in the ancient world were located at the Asclepian temple sites. At festival times, these were packed with audiences of pilgrims who combined a religious event with entertainment and fun.

The eighth and 18th days of each month were special for Asclepius and regular festivals were part of his celebration. At Athens, the festival of Asclepius took place on the day before the Great Dionysia (ET 560)[17]. Athenians also dedicated the fourth day of their mystic rites, associated with the worship of the Eleusinian goddesses Demeter and Persephone, to Asclepius. This part of the festival was named 'Epidauria' to commemorate Asclepius' arrival at Athens from Epidaurus in the form of a serpent in 420 BC[18]. Titane had twice-yearly festivals and Rome celebrated his 'birthday', ie the founding of his two temples, on 1 January and 11 September. The cities of Laodicea in Phrygia, Ancyra in Galatia, Tyre in Phoenicia, and Nicaea in Bithynia commemorated their festivals on coins with the inscription ΑϹΚΛΗΠΙΕΙΑ. The greatest festival occurred every four years at Epidaurus; it began nine days after the Isthmian Games and continued from April to June.

Poets, playwrights and actors competed for prizes at the festivals, where even physicians participated in medical competitions. These featured essays on treatment, diagnosis and surgical techniques, as well as demonstrations of new instrument designs. A record from Ephesus in Asia Minor describes a second or third century AD medical contest judged by a jury consisting of the priest of Asclepius and the presiding officer of the society of physicians. It was recorded that Vedius Rufinus won the essay prize, Aelius Meander the prize in surgery, and a contestant whose name is incomplete, Aelius ?, the prize for inventing new instruments (ET 573). Although the surname is missing, it is tempting to speculate that he was the same individual as the winner of the surgical award. This practice was the ancient equivalent of present-day Royal College of Physicians and Surgeons of Canada's annual awards for excellence in medical and surgical research or the various Scholar Awards of the American College of Physicians.

Stadia at Asclepian temples offered a variety of sporting spectacles, including activities conducive to mind–muscle coordination such as gymnastics, wrestling and boxing. The thrill of racing and an appetite for gambling was catered for by various competitions on both foot and horseback.

Many Asclepian temples enjoyed the right of sanctuary. This entitled a criminal, who reached the *cella* (central area of a temple) where the cult statue was located, to the right of asylum ie protection from the law. This tradition was adopted by the Romans and became part of Roman civil law. Even after Christianity became the official state religion, pagan temples retained this exclusive right and it was not until 399 AD that some Christian churches were granted the privilege.

Payment to the temple varied with the patient's ability to pay: the wealthy gave more to compensate for the poor who were treated without charge. The system resembles that of 'public ward care' and 'private patients' existing in hospitals before the introduction of government healthcare provision.

'Asclepius may heal Pauson and Iros [typical names of paupers in Greek comedy] and any one else who's hard up.' Aelianus, *Fragmenta*, 100 (ET 321)

'Euphanes, a boy from Epidaurus, suffering from stones, slept in the temple. It seemed to him the god stood by him and asked him: "What will you give me if I cure you?" "Ten dice," he answered. The god laughed and said he would cure him. When the day came he walked out fully recovered.' *Inscriptiones Graecae* IV, 1: 121–2 (ET 423)

Instructions to a wealthy patient included giving an Attic drachma to the bath attendant (ET 432). Pausanias in *Descriptio Graeciae*, X, 38, 13 (ET 444) reports the story of a wealthy blind man being handed a sealed tablet from Asclepius: '... he took away the seal, and when he looked at the wax he was cured, and he gave to Anyte [the messenger] the amount that was written on the tablet, two thousand *staters* of gold'.

This balanced billing allowed the temples to offer all their facilities to the poor and even to house them in guest accommodation. It was a fine example of social conscience, leading to the wealthy adopting a tradition of donating facilities for the poor. This seed may have germinated fully in the Christian era when the church catered to the poor and sick and provided hostels and poorhouses for them. In addition to making cash payments to the temple, healed patients contributed a votive of thanks depicting the diseased part or attesting to the cure received. Patients who defaulted on their payments had their cures reversed and were obliged to pay an additional penalty in order to regain favour.

The Asclepieia of Epidaurus, Cos and Pergamum developed ideal ancillary facilities for comprehensive healthcare which, even today, are not equalled by most major medical institutions.

Notes and references

1. The temples of the Olympian gods were temporary homes or their place of work. They lived on Mount Olympus.
2. Vitruvius (Marcus V Pollio). *De architectura*. Translated by Granger F. The Loeb Classical Library. Massachusetts: Harvard University Press, MCMLXXXV; Book VIII, chap 3: 151–79.
3. Jackson R. Waters and spas in the classical world. *Medical History* 1990; Suppl 10: 1–13.
4. Papadakis T. *Epidauros*. 7th edn. Munchen: Verlag Schnell & Steiner, 1988.
5. Kerenyi C. *Asklepios*. New York: Pantheon Books Inc, 1959.
6. Wedlake WJ. *The excavation of the shrine of Apollo at Nettleton 1956–1971*. Wiltshire: The Society of Antiquaries, 1982. Unfortunately, the excavators did not report on the presence or absence of snake bones.
7. The Medusa, chief of the Gorgons, was an appropriate decoration for his throne. Perseus struck off her head and Athena gave Asclepius some of her blood that had the power to raise the dead. The Chimera was a monster with a lion's head, a goat's body and a dragon's tail; the name is used in medicine today in order to refer to an individual, organ or part consisting of tissues of diverse genetic constitution.
8. Dogs had an association with Asclepius and Celtic healing deities; they also had a chthonian association with Cerberus, the three-headed dog that guarded the entrance to the infernal regions. The dogs shown with Asclepius were large, possibly reflecting the early association with Apollo Maleatas or hunter. A votive of an Irish wolfhound was found at the temple of Nodens, who was also a hunter deity (see [14]). Smaller dogs have been associated with female healing deities as at Coventina's Well on Hadrian's Wall and at the temple of Sulis Minerva in Bath.
9. The ancient plane tree under which Hippocrates is reputed to have taught still stands and receives intensive geriatric care from arborists and physicians. Any branches requiring amputation are carefully treated and preserved; they are then given to various medical associations that incorporate the wood into parts of their official regalia, such as the handle of the mace of the American College of Physicians.

10. Davaris D. *Kos: Hippocrates' island.* Translated by Heath M. Athens: Karydakis Bros, 1978.

11. Donaldson TL. *Ancient architecture.* Chicago: Argonaut Inc, 1965.

12. Gultekin H. *The askelepieion of Pergamon.* International edn. *Image Roche* 1965; **13**.

13. Edelstein EJ, Edelstein L. *Asclepius: interpretation of the testimonies.* Baltimore: Johns Hopkins Press, 1945: 191.

14. Wheeler REM, Wheeler TV. *Report of the prehistoric, Roman and post-Roman site in Lydney Park, Gloucestershire.* London: The Society of Antiquaries, 1932.

15. Walton A. *The cult of Asklepios.* New York: Ginn & Co for Cornell University Press, 1894. Reprinted by Johnson Reprint Corporation, New York and Johnson Reprint Co Ltd, London, 1965.

16. The description of Asclepius being unaffected by the passing of a large volume of wind from the bowels reveals the ancient appreciation for ethical behaviour. One of the hardest tasks for medical students to learn is to remain stoical and ignore the sounds and smell of the passage of flatus.

17. The Dionysia at Athens were a cultural event where new poets, actors and other artistes presented their work. The Roman Bacchanalia was not equivalent!

18. The Eleusinian Mysteries were special celebrations for Demeter. These took place at Eleusis and were later taken over by the Athenian state and held in Athens. The rites had to do with the initiates obtaining a happy life beyond the grave; these were kept secret and hence the name 'Mysteries'. Demeter forbade her followers to cultivate beans; this has a modern day explanation in that some people of Mediterranean origin suffer from an enzyme defect in their red blood cells. If persons with this glucose 6 phosphate dehydrogenase (G6PD) enzyme defect inhale or ingest certain compounds, their red blood cells undergo rapid destruction which results in acute haemolytic anaemia. Fava beans cause this in susceptible people. Pythagoras also forbade his followers to eat the fava bean. The Pythagoreans inhabited the south of Italy, the area that currently remains the world's highest incidence of G6PD enzyme deficiency.

Chapter 5

Asclepian temple medicine

Asclepian temple medicine served the needs of local inhabitants as well as pilgrims from far away places. Supplicant needs varied from the simple to the complex. Some came to thank Asclepius or to pray for the relief of minor symptoms and continuing health, while others had prolonged visits in order to cure more serious illnesses and to undergo 'incubation'[1]. Temple treatment evolved from an emphasis solely on the nootherapy (mind therapy) of the sixth to fifth centuries BC to the added provision of actual medical treatment. Physicians who did not take part in any of the temple rituals offered their services to supplicants outside the temple precinct.

Temple priests: noology and theurgy

Asclepius priests practised noology, a philosophy based on the belief that illness was due to imbalances in the body. When the mind becomes harmonious with nature, the imbalances are corrected and health is restored. Priests and early Greek philosophers had the earliest explanation for the relationship between *psyche* and *soma*. Plato believed that health was the only natural condition of man and that it could be disturbed by morbid, internal disharmonies. This philosophy was partially described in *The Symposium* where Plato's hypothetical physician, Eryximachus, states that the most skilful doctor is one who must be able to '...bring elements in the body which are most hostile to one another into a happy and loving relationship; such hostile elements are the opposites: cold and hot; bitter and sweet; dry and wet and the like. It was by knowing how to promote love and harmony between these, as our two poets here say and as I believe, that our forefather Asclepius founded our science'[2]. This philosophical theory of balancing qualities in the body, formulated in the fifth century BC by Empedocles of Acragas in Sicily, became the physiological basis for the humoral theory of disease, which remained the basis of medical thinking until the Renaissance (see chapter 8).

Restoration of health by the mind required 'the purity of thought' which supplicants were admonished to acquire when they passed under the inscription on the propylaea of the sanctuary of Asclepius at

Epidaurus. Purity of thought resulted not only in thinking 'holy thoughts' but also required the abolition of dissatisfaction, envy, anger, insecurity and psychoneuroses. Shedding unpleasant and unhealthy thoughts was, and still is, assisted by a variety of activities and distractions dispelling introversion. The philosopher-priests of Asclepius understood the influence of mental stress on physical disease — the ambience of their temples helped calm the mind and bring back mental harmony. When patients contemplated the beauty of the temple's surroundings and its aesthetic architecture, there was a diminution of imbalanced thoughts. Beautiful landscapes still have the power to do this but most of today's psychiatric hospitals do not have the facilities enjoyed by supplicants at the Asclepian sanctuaries.

Facilities for appreciation of the rhythm of music, dance and poetry calmed the soul and encouraged the use of music to create internal harmony. An awakened appreciation of music enhanced the enjoyment of hymn singing at temple services and supplicants may have started to hum melodies, giving praise to Asclepius and joy for themselves. Temple theatres featured tragedies resulting in a therapeutic catharsis of the emotions, and comedies which lessened their inner tensions and produced a sense of wellbeing. These various pleasurable pursuits provided opportunities for social interaction between fellow supplicants, reducing the significance of their illnesses, and allowed their minds to strive for ideals and purity. Today, a similar therapeutic innovation exists called 'group therapy'.

Dedications and votives proclaiming successful cure were displayed in prominent places throughout temple compounds. Supplicants identified testimonials of cure relating to conditions similar to their own and this aura of successful treatment infused powerful reassurance for an optimistic outcome of their own temple stay.

Entry into the *abaton*, with its nocturnal ceremonies, was restricted to those undergoing 'incubation'. This exclusion enhanced the mystery of visits by Asclepius during temple sleep so it was anticipated with enthusiasm; supplicants entered with a pre-conditioned mood for a successful outcome.

The infrastructure necessary for successful temple therapy required ancillary facilities for music, theatre, exercise, social discourse, and accommodation facilities.

Incubation
The climax of treatment by priests was the 'incubation' or ritual temple sleep. Psychological conditioning (nootherapy) and a suitable period of conservative therapy (discussed below) preceded the theurgical cure.

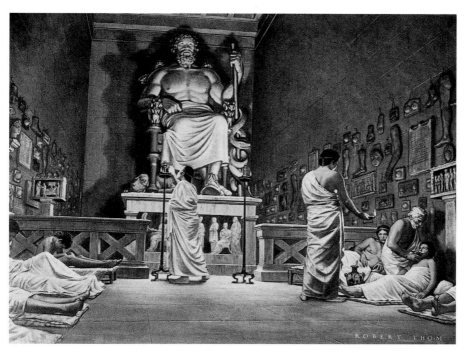

Figure 37 Artistic depiction of the temple sleep or 'incubation' ritual (Photo courtesy Parke-Davis Co, Scarborough, ON, Canada (Great Moments in Medicine))

Some temples provided a special *abaton* where entry was forbidden to the non-initiated and those who had not completed the preliminary purification ceremonies necessary for the appearance of the god. The most sacred *abaton* was the adytum, however, the precise role of this facility still remains unknown. Not all patients slept in the *abaton* — this area may have been the ancient counterpart of a 'private patients pavilion'. At many sanctuaries, supplicants slept in the portico, anteroom or on the floor where men, who used the eastern portion, were separated from women in the west. Before their ritual sleep, patients purified themselves by bathing in cold water and were dressed in white as, by tradition, this was thought to favour dreams. They brought their own bedding and sacrificial cakes flavoured with wine or honey; it is possible that supplicants were given a preceding potion to help them sleep and promote dreams. The *abaton* was kept in semi-darkness and flickering lights from perfumed candles and lamps accentuated the majestic 'cult statue' of Asclepius (Figure 37). The priests and priestesses, with their hair bound in white fillets, dressed like Asclepius and Hygieia with Egyptian sandals on their feet and circulated among the sleepers with their serpents and dogs. This was the time of magical cures when supplicants dreamt that Asclepius had visited and cured them by performing surgery, manipulation or providing a prescription. This 'treatment' by Asclepius was so gentle that the patient was not awakened; perhaps this is what is referred to by the dedication to Asclepius on the altar at Chester, inscribed 'Asclepius of the gentle hands' (chapter 7; Figure 60). The reality of the supplicants' dreams was augmented by the priests touching them and by the serpents or dogs licking them, especially if some of the honey-flavoured cakes were nearby. The resulting slight disturbance to their sleep would reaffirm their belief in a visit by Asclepius, just as today when sleeping children hear their parents on Christmas Eve and believe they have heard Father Christmas.

The dreams patients experienced often reflected their own attitudes to their illness and their aspirations for cure. Some patients credited their cure to exaggerated and grotesque surgery being a simplistic interpretation of their treatment. For instance:

'Arata, a woman of Lacedaemon (Sparta), was dropsical. While she remained in Lacedaemon, her mother slept in the temple on her behalf and saw a dream. It seemed to her that the god cut off her daughter's head and hung up her body in such a way that her throat was turned downwards. Out of it came a huge amount of fluid. He then took down the body and fitted her head back onto her neck. After she had seen this dream she went back to Lacedaemon where she found her daughter in good health; she had seen the same dream.' *Inscriptiones Graecae* IV, 1, 121–2, Stele I Cures of Apollo and Asclepius (ET 423)

Several dream-cures involved surgery on the abdomen, a procedure not practised at that time apart from drainage of a liver abscess. Some of the dream prescriptions have been recorded:

'There is, I believe, a compound of Philo's. I could not even smell it before, but when the god gave me a sign to use it and also signified the time at which it was necessary to do this, not only did I drink it easily, but, as soon as I drank it, I immediately felt happier and better. What is more, it would be possible to say ten thousand other things about drugs — some of which he himself compounded, others belonging to the common or garden varieties which he prescribed as a cure for the body, as appropriate in each individual case.' (Aristides, *Oratio* XLIX, 29–30) (ET 410)

Another remedy of interest was described by the Elder Pliny, *Natural History*, XXV, 4(11), (30) (ET 369):

'The most effective remedies for diseases of the rectum are wool-grease . . . the ashes of a dog's head; the sloughed skin of a serpent, with vinegar. In cases where there is chapping, the ashes of the white portions of dogs' excreta, mixed with oil of roses; they say that this is an invention of Asclepius and that by the same treatment warts are most easily removed.'[3]

One dream prescription showed a sense of humour and practicality; Asclepius prescribed a diet of excess pork for the treatment of haemoptysis (blood spitting) and, when asked what he would have done if the patient were Jewish, he replied that he would recommend another prescription (ET 427).

If a patient had not dreamt specifically of cure by Asclepius, then he would report his dreams to the priest who interpreted them and prescribed some form of therapy. Priests' recommendations seem today like a mixture of traditional remedies and folklore combined with imagination and common sense. Although many patients suffered from untreatable illnesses, it was very likely that they benefited from the nootherapy[4]. They may also have received some form of placebo effect during their stay, with a temporary improvement of their illness[5]. Patients had great faith in Asclepius and the incubation ritual was a dramatic culmination to their temple visit. It gave conditioned patients the ultimate placebo effect as well as psychological reinforcement to their positive thinking and self-cure. As a result of their temple visit, patients paid more attention to their health and became more compliant with their doctor's care. Galen described this in *Commentarius in Hippocratis Epidemias* (VI iv, Sectio IV, 8):

' . . . even among ourselves in Pergamum we see that those being treated by the god obey him when he orders them, as he does on many occasions, not to drink at all for 15 days, while they obey none of the physicians who give this prescription. For a patient will really be encouraged to do everything that is prescribed if he or she has been strongly persuaded that he will gain real benefit from doing so.' (ET 401)

Patients may have been worried about the prospect of the solemn incubation ceremony. Attendance at the temple theatre featuring humorous plays may have relieved some of this tension. An entertaining, if irreverent portrayal, of incubation survives in the satirical comic play *Plutus* by Aristophanes lines 653–758 (abridged) (chapter 4) (ET 420) :

'Cario: Soon we got to the God's temple, bringing poor old Plutus with us. He wasn't in good shape then, but it's a different story now! First we took him to the sea and gave him a bath.

Plutus' wife: What a lucky chap! So the poor old fellow had a dip in the ice-cold sea?

Cario: Then we went to the sacred precinct of the God. On the altar we offered wheat cakes and other items to the flames of Hephaestus. There we lay Plutus down just as they normally do. We each stitched up a mattress for ourselves.

Plutus' wife: Were there others waiting to be cured?

Cario: ... There were many people there, sick with every kind of disease. Soon, the man in charge put out the lights and told us to go to sleep. We were told not to get up or to speak, whatever noise we heard. So down we lay resting quietly. ... The God went round to every patient, treading calmly and quietly, examining his or her disease. Then by his side a slave put a stone pestle and mortar and a medicine chest. First of all he mixed up a plaster for Neoclides [an unpopular figure in Athens at that time], throwing in three cloves of Tenian garlic. With these he mixed sour grape juice and sea onions. He beat them up together and poured vinegar from Sphettus onto them. Then turning up the man's eyelids, he plastered the inner sides to make it more uncomfortable; this made him jump up yelling and shouting and he tried to run away. ... Then after that he sat down beside Plutus. First, he felt the patient's head then he took a linen napkin, clean and white, wiped both his eyelids and made them dry. Then Panacea, with a scarlet coloured cloth covered up his face and head. Then the God made animal noises and out of the temple came two gi-normous serpents.

Plutus' wife: Ye gods!

Cario: And they crept underneath the scarlet cloth and licked his eyelids, so it seemed. And madam, before you could have drunk ten cups of wine, Plutus got up and he could see once more!'

Conservative (expectant) therapy

Divine serendipity helped in the success of Asclepian temple medicine. The preparation of patients for the incubation ritual, and the ancillary facilities developed for nootherapy, provided the same essential elements as those of 20th century conservative, or expectant, therapy.

This was the mainstay of medical treatment before the 'wonder-drug era' of the 1950s. Conservative therapy uses the techniques of adequate rest and relaxation, controlled diet, effective elimination, and exercise combined with reassurance and tincture of time. Many common conditions continue to respond to this routine which completely avoids the complications of medications, invasive procedures and surgery.

Temples were ideal locations for rest and relaxation and their beautiful architecture and location equalled any of our present-day luxury 'country house hotels'. Priests controlled the preparation time for the incubation ceremony, including an assessment of the duration of rest and relaxation needed. Such a technique resembles the physician's assessment of the amount of rest prescribed for a heart attack in the 1950s. Rest continues to be the mainstay of treatment for a variety of conditions ranging from sprains, fractures and contusions to infections, cardiovascular, neurological, arthritic and gastrointestinal diseases. Removal of the psychological and mental stresses of daily living is healthy for the mind and accompanying psychoneurotic symptoms.

Asclepius advocated a simple diet and did not treat diseases caused by gluttony and other excesses. This policy was outlined by Philostratus in *Vita Apollonii*, I, 9 (ET 397) describing an Assyrian youth who, after a life of luxury and drunkenness (substance abuse), was suffering from dropsy (fluid swelling of the body) and had been refused treatment by Asclepius:

'For he gives [health] to those who want it, but you do things that make your disease worse, for you give yourself up to luxury, and go on piling a rich diet onto your water-logged and worn out innards as if you were clogging up water with a load of mud.'

This is a good description of an alcoholic with ascites (fluid in the abdominal cavity) and generalized oedema (soft swelling which pits on pressure). Asclepius was the first physician to become exasperated by noncompliant alcoholic patients but many subsequent physicians have shared his frustrations! The simple diets of the Asclepieia may have had a high fibre content which would relieve a variety of gastrointestinal symptoms. This theory is supported by Aristides, *Oratio* XLIX, 28 (ET 411), who wrote: 'Again, he told me to eat the same drug together with wheat-bread, which I ate near the holy tripod, and I then started on the road to recovery'.

A simple diet combined with high fluid intake and tincture of time would treat some symptoms of lead poisoning. In the Roman world, plumbism was a common complication of peace and prosperity. This was not due to lead plumbing but caused by lead used as an ingredient for sweetening agents in food and wine[6]. In the preparation of wine, *defrutum* (must) was prepared by evaporating fruit juices in a lead-containing pewter or lead-glazed vessel. The acid juices leeched lead from the container, resulting in a sweeter flavour to the residual fluid. A simple diet would have removed this common source of lead ingestion and, when combined with waters from the temple spring, would have lowered blood lead levels and reduced abdominal cramps, weakness and other symptoms of lead intoxication.

The Athenian association of Asclepius with the goddesses Demeter and Persephone probably resulted in the exclusion of beans from the diet. Other benefits of a simple but balanced diet are weight loss, reduction of blood lipids and blood sugar as well as correction of vitamin deficiencies. Patients avoided excess wine, which may have helped relieve attacks of gout, but this was also used as a vehicle for drugs and was prescribed for its convalescent properties as shown on a coin of Pergamum depicting Telesphorus holding a bunch of grapes (Figure 16).

Ritual drinking of the temple spring waters provided more benefit than just cleansing the soul. A high fluid intake flushed the body's system and helped constipation. Minerals present in some of the springs had a cathartic effect and may have been useful in the treatment of other disorders. Spring waters would have reduced the need for purging, and it is likely there were specialized facilities for treatment by clyster (enema).

The location of temples encouraged the desire for walking, which is one of the most effective forms of exercise. At the gymnasia and stadia, patients followed a discipline of coordinated movements and were encouraged into skilful and competitive physical activities. Galen wrote about exercise in *De Sanitate Tuenda* (Keeping Healthy) I, 8, 19–21 (ET 413) and said: '. . . our ancestral god Asclepius . . . ordered hunting and horse riding and exercising in arms . . . For he not only desired to awake a lust for life in those who were apathetic, but also outlined ways in which this could be achieved in the form of exercises'. This physical activity eliminated feelings of aggression and increased the strength of mind and body. These activities were the ancient counterpart of today's aerobic exercises where exercise has been rediscovered as a valuable adjunct for a healthy body. Carefully controlled vigorous exercise is good for the cardiovascular system and has been shown to release hormones (endomorphins) which result in a psychological high. It is part of the rehabilitation programme for fractures and locomotor disorders and injuries. The baths would have provided facilities for swimming and sudotherapy, and at sites having hot springs there were the added benefits of whirlpool massage[7] which aids recovery from injuries to muscles, tendons, soft tissues and joints. The gymnasia and baths of the Asclepieia resembled the exercise rooms and health spas of present-day health clubs and hotels.

Reassurance is an essential component of conservative therapy. The patient needs to have a positive attitude and confidence about recovery but should also realize that time is required and must not become impatient. All this was accomplished by the facilities and diversions of the temple already described. Even today, more than one Harley Street specialist in London has prescribed the West-end theatres, walking trips to Harrods or Bond Street and visits to the casinos as an ancillary aid in the treatment of wealthy patients from abroad. Votives and testimonials from cured patients were displayed in prominent parts of the temple complex and even decorated the walls of the *abaton*. The sick derived strong doses of hope and optimism from the votives depicting the diseased parts of cured patients, as well as from the written testimonies of prominent citizens. In medicine today, we are now rediscovering the value of positive thinking and hope; in the antibiotic and 'wonder-drug' era of the 1950s to 1970s, positive thinking was not emphasized and was replaced by prescriptions which were frequently inappropriate and had potentially adverse side-effects. The most common example of this was the custom of prescribing penicillin for viral infections and the development of penicillin sensitivity. In her book *Imagery in healing: shamanism and modern medicine*, Achterberg reviews the therapeutic value of the cult of Aesculapius and of native doctors and shamans[8]. Her work is supported by references to a variety of controlled clinical studies including one which assesses the response of children with acute leukaemia undergoing chemotherapy; those who positively imaged destruction of the 'bad' cells fared better than a control group. The value of the 'placebo effect' is still doubted by some physicians and is thought to be a ploy for patients with psychological disease. Experienced oncologists know the therapeutic advantage of a positive attitude in effecting the results of their treatment; even making a return appointment for a dying patient gives a ray of hope and often results in proving the immediate prognosis wrong. This is the true art of medicine which may assist the outcome of many diseases. Dr Ian Stevenson, Professor of Psychiatry at the University of Virginia Medical School, wrote an article 'Preserving the healing power of hope'[9] which described the shattering effect on the wellbeing of a patient treated with cold science without the benefit of hope and the art of medicine. The patient was his wife!

Temple visits for 'inpatients' often required a sojourn of several weeks and this allowed for action of the tincture of time. Some of the larger temples provided guest accommodation but this was limited and patients often had to stay at facilities nearby. In reality, the patient had a holiday with a break from daily responsibilities and with ample opportunity for physical and mental rest, factors still facilitating recovery from many physical and mental illnesses. The awareness of time in healing is recorded in the thank-offering to Asclepius by the Athenian orator, Aeschines (ET 404): 'I had despaired of the skill of mortals, but had placed every hope in the divine... I came to your sacred grove, Asclepius, and I was healed in three months of a festering wound which I had had on my head for a whole year.'

Until very recently, such wounds would require many weeks of local treatment before they healed.

Summary
The achievements of Asclepian temple medicine were remarkable. They focused attention on health and dispensed reassurance to patients. They marshalled the powers of positive thinking and assisted the body's repair and immune systems. By serendipity, temple sojourns resulted in optimal conservative therapy, and their facilities for total mental care were not equalled until this century. The exhibited anatomical votives gave reassurance resulting in supplicants positively imaging their own diseased parts[10]. During the incubation ritual, patients dreamt they had been treated by Asclepius although, in reality, had been touched by either a temple priest, serpent or dog — the pre-conditions were such that significant cure or healing was often achieved. Even today, participation in care by non-divine 'healers' has been considered to be one of numerous and miscellaneous techniques that help patients by caring efforts[11].

Patients visiting the temples had conditions either liable to respond to conservative therapy and spontaneous recovery or were psychosomatic in origin. Travel time to the temples would exclude patients with acute infections and terminal illnesses. The exclusion of those women about to deliver also eliminated foetal and neonatal mortality. Therefore, any statistical analysis of response rate would use patient samples slanted towards those who would recover and supplicants did not represent a random selection of patients. Even those suffering from chronic disorders were candidates for temporary relief from a variety of measures giving a placebo effect.

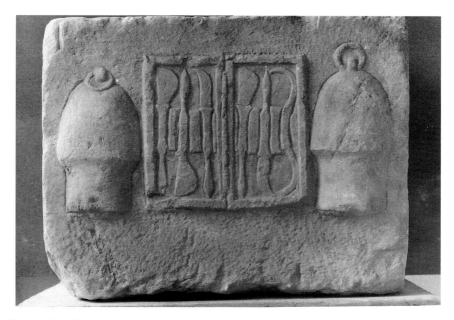

Figure 38   Bas-relief on the tombstone of a physician at the Asclepieion of Athens, depicting a case of surgical instruments flanked by cupping vessels (Photo National Archaeological Museum of Greece, Athens)

After the fourth century BC, physicians became associated with temple medicine (see chapter 8). A tombstone, found in the Asclepieion of Athens, depicted a case of surgical instruments and a cupping vessel (Figure 38). Without an existing liaison, it is likely that the temple authorities would not have permitted this display of the familiar tools of the physician.

Notes and references

1. Hospitals treat inpatients and outpatients. This division could be applied to temple medicine with those undergoing the incubation ritual being considered inpatients. In view of the large number of patients and the limited facilities, control of patient flow was essential and it is possible some type of 'advanced booking' was made for the incubation ritual.
2. Plato. *The Symposium*. Translated by Hamilton W. London: Penguin Books, 1951.
3. Warts have been charmed away by a variety of methods. I was suspicious of some of my dermatology teacher's statements in this regard and conducted a few clinical trials on my friends' children. Faith in the doctor figure was important. My therapeutic tool was a 1927 Indian-head American nickel that had been smoked over an old alcohol spirit lamp. The carbon was then rubbed on the wart and was not to be washed off for a week. Perhaps the warts were due to disappear anyway but it was a painless form of therapy. I do not plan to conduct a controlled therapeutic trial using white dog dung!

4. Palliative care helps patients with incurable diseases. The patient's environment is made as pleasing and comfortable as possible, and care providers provide personal attention to their physical and emotional needs. This results in less pain and allows patients to enjoy their remaining time to the fullest.

5. Placebo effect is experienced by advanced cancer patients who travel to distant clinics to try unproven remedies. These patients feel better during their short stay at the clinic but deteriorate rapidly when they return home.

6. Farwell DE, Molleson TL. *Excavations at Poundbury 1966–80. Volume II: The cemeteries*. Dorset Natural History and Archaeological Society, Monograph Series, 1993, No 11.

7. The entry of hot spring water into the ancient baths was similar to the hot water jets of a jacuzzi or whirlpool bath.

8. Achterberg J. *Imagery in healing: shamanism and modern medicine*. New Science Library, 1985.

9. Stevenson I. Preserving the healing power of hope. *Pharos* (publication of the AOA Honour Medical Society), Summer 1984.

10. The positive role of imaging in the modern treatment of heart disease has been studied by Dr Dean Ornish and is a component of his therapy for reversing heart disease. New York Times bestseller book: *Dr Dean Ornish's program for reversing heart disease*. New York: Ballantine Books, 1996.

11. Lane Fox R. Healing powers. *J R Soc Med* 1998; **91**(4): 177.

Chapter 6

Votives and talismans

Votives

Votives were a special form of remuneration given to the gods for their services to mankind. When a supplicant had vowed to give a particular payment in return for having a request fulfilled, the gift became an ex voto. Votives were made from a variety of materials, but all were designed to please the god or provide an appropriate indication of appreciation. They took various forms, including anatomical models of body parts, tools, weapons and figurines, as well as dedications and written testimonies. For some gods, votives were intentionally bent or broken at the time of giving; this practice indicated that the gift was intended solely for the god and not to be used by others. Such votive bending, however, was not practised at Asclepian temples as the display of gifts from cured patients generated hope and confidence among those seeking treatment. Today, preserved specimens continue to commemorate healing and reflect the spectrum of ailments treated. The study of ordinary anatomical votives gives a general depiction of the ailments suffered by the donors whereas custom votives provide accurate details, allowing precise diagnosis.

Anatomical votives

Anatomical votives, depicting diseased areas of the body, were given to the various healing deities of the ancient world. They were mass-produced locally from wood, stone, clay or metal, and were sold at the Asclepieia from stalls or shops in the temple compound. Votives of the extremities were frequently pierced to facilitate wall display, while votive heads and torso parts featured a flat base for exhibition on shelves and tables. All votives at the Asclepieia were considered to be the sacred property of Asclepius and could not be destroyed or recycled. Those that accumulated in excess were buried in sacred pits dug in the temple compound; occasionally, as at Athens, an inscription was made recording these superfluous objects. Some votives were thrown into springs, wells, lakes, rivers and ponds that were sacred to water deities. Archaeologists have recovered thousands of votives,

providing us with an outstanding record of diseases treated at the
sanctuaries of healing gods.

At Ponte di Nona, situated east of Rome, 8,000 votives were
excavated from a sanctuary that served an ancient farming community[1]. Two-thirds of these depicted arms, hands, legs or feet; there
were four times as many models of feet than there were of hands.
Although none of the votives showed specific disease, the frequency of
those depicting feet reflects the pedestrian nature of farm life which
involved much walking on uneven ground with poor protective
footwear. Symptoms arising from infection, arthritis or injury of the
feet would have curtailed the sufferer's livelihood.

Several votive heads were also found at Ponte di Nona; these are
thought to be associated with headache. In 1988, Jackson speculated
that the frequency of headache at this site may have been related to the
local prevalence of malaria[1]. Many votive eyes were found, some
depicting the eye alone and others with its lids and periocular tissue;
Jackson suggested this represented an attempt to depict eye disease
separately from disease of the lids and periocular tissues (trachoma)
which were common in antiquity[1]. Few votives of genitalia occurred,
proposing that either such problems were uncommon at Ponte di Nona
or the sanctuary did not attempt to cure them.

Hundreds of votives have been found at Corinth. Most of these
depict arms and hands, legs and feet, but there are also 18
representatives of complete male genitalia[2]. Other temples have
revealed numerous votives of male or female genitalia; most are likely
to be gifts for the cure of common genitourinary complaints but some
may also express gratitude for the birth of a child. Only three eye
votives were found at this site, although many more were found at
Wroxeter and Athens. This may indicate that either eye diseases were
rare at Corinth or other centres specialized in ophthalmic treatment.
Replica eyes and ears were common and used to indicate disease; they
were also used as a supplication for the donor to be seen or heard by
Asclepius.

Archaeological findings from Viroconium (Wroxeter), cantonal
capital of Cornovii (now considered to be the fourth largest town of
Roman Britain), suggest this site may have been an ophthalmic centre.
Excavations in the basilica debris revealed more than 100 votive eyes
modelled from wall plaster [personal communication, Dr RH White,
University of Birmingham] (Figure 39). These vary in style, detail and
size and were produced individually. They were not pierced for
suspension or display and their size is such that they can be held in the
palm of the hand. The medical significance of the plaster eyes is

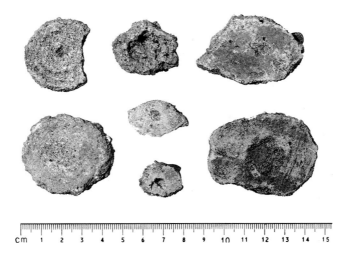

Figure 39 Sample from the many votive eyes found at Wroxeter, dating to the second or third century AD. These were made from plaster with anatomical details varying from being barely recognizable to the central votive which clearly demonstrates the pupil and lower lid as well as the inner and outer canthus (Photo by Sidney C Renow, Esher, Surrey; kindly supplied by Dr Roger White, Shrewsbury and Wroxeter Museums, Shropshire, England)

enhanced by the finding of a representation pair of eyes made from beaten gold and another in bronze[3]. By contrast, there were no votives depicting other body parts. This is unique archaeological evidence for the presence of a deity specializing in the treatment of eye diseases.

The finding of two oculist's stamps and a set of medical instruments are strong evidence for concurrent medical therapy. One oculist's stamp, found at Wroxeter in 1808, is circular with the inscription: 'The dialibanum of Tiberius Claudius, the physician, for all complaints of the eyes, to be used with egg' (dialibanum was an aromatic medication made from frankincense)[4,5]. The second stamp, found in 1981, indicated that it belonged to 'Q...Lucillianus' but, unfortunately, further details about its use were not included[6]. Not only were these stamps used to label the 'prescription' of an eye ointment, they also identified two Roman eye specialists (*medici ocularii*) at Wroxeter.

A case of surgical instruments, found in a grave at the cemetery north of Wroxeter in 1862, provides further evidence for medical treatment in this town. The surgical lancet had remained in such good condition that a 19th century physician remarked that he would still be able to use it! This instrument was originally stored in a wooden box that also contained '... some beads, a portion of a needle or bodkin, which had somewhat the appearance of a handle of a small spoon, other fragments of metal and the remains of two very small earthenware vessels, containing a very hard substance resembling white dried paint'[4]. This description teases the imagination. Could the 'needle or bodkin' be similar to the handled needle, complete with screw-thread cover, which had been used for cataract operations and was found at Corbridge? Might the 'white dried paint' be an eye ointment such as that described by the Elder Pliny as containing white zinc oxide[7]?

Roman physicians at Wroxeter were probably either *medici* associated with the legionary fortress that preceded the civilian town, or physicians who had set up civilian practice locally after their discharge from the army. The hospital associated with the legionary fortress remains to be found; two temple sites have been located at Wroxeter, however, neither has been excavated. A definitive explanation for the eyes must, therefore, await future archaeological findings. Excavations undertaken in the town of Wroxeter have uncovered depictions in stone or bronze of eight different deities; one of these was Apollo, a healing deity in the Celtic world[8] and who was associated with light and, thus, sight. Apollo's later association with light, in addition to his other responsibilities, would suggest an additional reason for invoking this particular deity.

In addition to Wroxeter, the Athenian Asclepieion had a preponderance of eye votives; at Epidaurus, there were frequent testimonies to blindness and other eye diseases. Findings of many clusters of votives depicting lungs, ribs, uteri, heads and breasts at other sites may also indicate specialized interests and practice. Some depict the organs of the female pelvis and one in the Drake Collection of the Canadian Museum of Health and Medicine depicts a bicornate uterus.

Custom votives

Although most anatomical votives were mass-produced, the wealthy could afford custom designed replicas that portrayed exact details of the diseased part. Accurate depictions of the cured affliction were certain to please the healing deities. Today, these artefacts are an invaluable aid to diagnosing the nature of disease in antiquity.

The votive leg in Figure 40a provides an excellent depiction of varicosities on the long saphenous vein and contrasts significantly with the mass-produced, terracotta leg shown in Figure 40b which does not allow diagnosis. Patients with varicose veins experience two complications likely to respond well to Asclepian temple medicine. The most common is superficial inflammation of the vein (thrombophlebitis), a

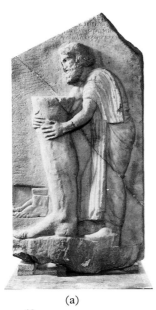

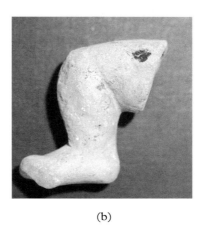

(b)

(a)

Figure 40
(a) Custom votive of a leg depicting varicosities in the long saphenous vein (larger than life-size) (Photo National Archaeological Museum, Athens, Greece)
(b) Mass-produced votive leg, either a child's or an obese adult, with crude style and details (10 cm). It might even depict swelling but the lack of detail precludes making a diagnosis (GDH)

non-fatal problem caused by factors such as prolonged standing or sitting, local pressure and stressful, unaccustomed exercise. It usually improves spontaneously with bed rest after about two weeks. The other complication that occurs with long-standing varicose veins is development of a varicose ulcer. This develops in poorly vascularized areas of the lower leg and becomes infected. Treatment involves a long period of rest, good general health measures and local antiseptic dressings — the Asclepieion was an ideal place for such treatment.

A terracotta votive reputed to have originated from the Asclepieion at Cos demonstrates a unique example of disease. This shows a young boy with a protuberant left eye (exophthalmos and proptosis) and a verrucous lesion on the left cheek; he is pursing his lips and appears to be puffing his cheeks (Figure 41a). This artefact, lost following World War Two, was in the Meyer-Steineg Collection at the University of Jena and was described in 1912 by Meyer-Steineg as depicting malignancy of the eye socket (sarcoma orbitae)[9]. More recent clinical studies of similar lesions of the orbit and neighbouring structures have been reported by McCord et al in 1968[10] and Lloyd et al in 1971[11,12]; these have led to the recognition of congenital abnormalities of eye

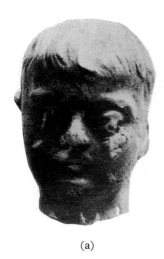
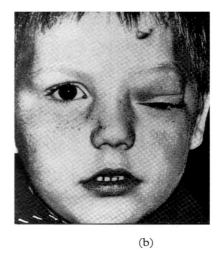

(a)   (b)

Figure 41
(a) Votive head from Cos depicting exophthalmos and lesion on cheek (Photo Prof
Dr G Zinserling, Archaeologisches Institute, University of Jena, Germany)
(b) A boy patient of the 1970s with orbital varices and a varicosity on the forehead
(Photo courtesy Dr GAS Lloyd and the *British Journal of Ophthalmology*, London,
England)

socket veins as a cause of intermittent, unilateral exophthalmos. The
degree of protrusion can be accentuated by increased pressure in the
veins of the orbit by activities such as bending forward, compressing
the neck, or performing the Valsalva manoeuvre (exhaling against
pursed lips). Dilated veins elsewhere in the head or body may
accompany the condition; protrusion of the orbit may be intermittent
in nature due to temporary blockage of a vein by a clot.

Orbital varices (distended, tortuous veins of the eye socket) are ideal
for apparent cure by Asclepian temple medicine. At the temple, natural
processes would recanalize the blocked vein and relieve the increased
venous pressure. Temple physicians or priests might have observed
that patients could aggravate the condition by performing the Valsalva
manoeuvre and would have instructed them not to do so as part of the
treatment. Figure 41a depicts the same lesions as shown in the modern
patient (Figure 41b).

An ivory ex voto depicting two flat breasts was found in the bath of
the temple of Sulis Minerva (Minerva Medica) at Bath, England
(Figure 42). Lindsay Allison-Jones suggested it to be a thanks-offering
for curing a common breast disease[13]. However, as most common
breast diseases produce swelling and the artist depicted two underdeveloped breasts, an alternative and more likely explanation for this

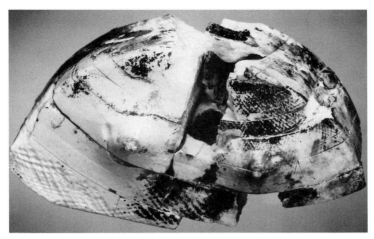

Figure 42   Votive made from ivory depicting small, flat breasts, found at the Roman Baths at Bath (Photo courtesy Ms Jane Bircher and © Roman Baths Museum, Bath, England)

votive is that it was given by a young woman with very small breasts who wished to improve her womanly figure. As there were no plastic surgeons in Bath in the second century AD, she sought the help of Minerva Medica to undergo augmentation mammoplasty achieved by divine means. It is probable that the votive was thrown into the sacred waters to draw attention to her wish.

Many votives and coins were recovered from the temple of Nodens at Lydney, England. Nodens was an Asclepian-style temple built in the late fourth century AD amid beautiful, wooded surroundings above disused Roman iron-workings. The complex includes, in addition to the temple itself, an *abaton*, shops, accommodation facilities, baths and reservoirs. One of the most intriguing finds is a bronze arm, terminating in a carefully detailed hand that may originally have held a round object[14]. The fingernails are exceptionally well sculpted and demonstrate a finding of great interest to haematologists: the nails are concave in both longitudinal and transverse axes (Figure 43). This deformity is called koilonychia, or spoon-shaped nails, and is a manifestation of severe iron deficiency. If a patient with such deficiency attended the temple at Lydney, and if part of the healing ritual was similar to that employed at other Asclepian sites in the ancient world, then healing would involve ingestion of the local, iron-rich water. The site includes the only intact shaft of a Roman iron mine and even today rusty water still drips from its ceiling (Plan 4, chapter 4). This water would have had a mystical appeal and contains adequate iron to treat koilonychia effectively, provided a prolonged stay in the guest house

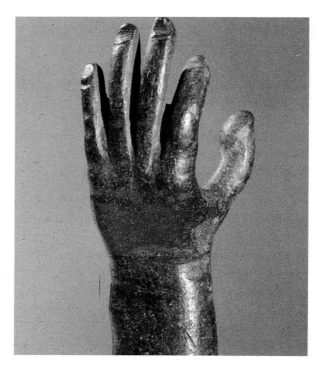

Figure 43 Bronze votive hand (25 mm long) showing spoon-shaped nails (koilonychiae) (Photo kindly supplied by Viscount Bledisloe of Lydney Park Museum, Gloucestershire, England)

accommodation was prescribed. After correction of the iron deficiency, the patient would have felt better and his or her nails grown back normally. A hand depicting koilonychia is the votive *par excellence* for severe iron deficiency[15].

A Graeco-Roman terracotta votive from the Drake Collection in the Canadian Museum of Health and Medicine depicts a bicornate uterus (Figure 44). This birth defect (congenital anomaly) occurs during embryonic development and is caused by incomplete fusion of the paired Müllerian ducts. It results in the development of a double womb (a variable degree of double uterus and a double cervix); the altered cavity of the womb causes miscarriage, while the altered opening results in difficult labour. Although a rare condition in women, it represents the normal anatomy of all female domestic animals. It is likely that the clay modeller producing this votive based his anatomical knowledge on animal examples. Thus, this votive may signify either a sophisticated obstetrical procedure or an old wives' tale.

In Roman times, midwives delivered most babies but specialist physicians were consulted for difficult labours. Soranus, the ancient

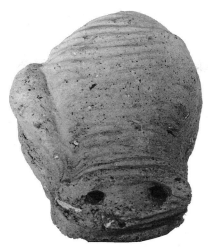

Figure 44   Terracotta Greek votive (third to first century BC) depicting a bicornate uterus with double cervix and ?fallopian tube (Photo © The Toronto Hospital and supplied by Felicity Pope, Curator of the Canadian Museum of Health and Medicine, Toronto, ON, Canada)

authority on obstetrics, advised physicians to listen carefully to the patient's case history as described by the midwife [personal communication, L Allison-Jones][16]. If she told the doctor that her patient had a history of miscarriages and was experiencing unexplained difficulties with labour, an experienced practitioner might suspect and diagnose a bicornate uterus. He would then select the cervical opening most suitable for manipulating the position of the foetus to pass through the uterus. A viable baby and mother in such circumstances would certainly merit a gift to Asclepius from both the doctor and the patient!

An alternative explanation for the votive is the common belief before 1950 that 'twins come from a double uterus'[17]. When twins were born, the joyous parents might aptly express their thanks by giving a custom-made votive based on the uterus of a domestic animal. This votive is an excellent example of this; the roll of tissue depicted on one side suggests that its manufacturer worked from an animal uterus which had been removed with one fallopian tube still attached.

The donation of anatomical votives to the deities at healing centres was not restricted to Asclepius. A unique, bronze votive was found at the shrine of Mercury at Uley in Gloucestershire, England. This is the miniature reproduction of a leg with reverse flexion at the knee joint or *genu recurvatum* (back knee), a rare condition that causes the foot to appear reversed (Figure 45)[18–20]. This orthopaedic condition results from congenital absence of the patella or congenital subluxation

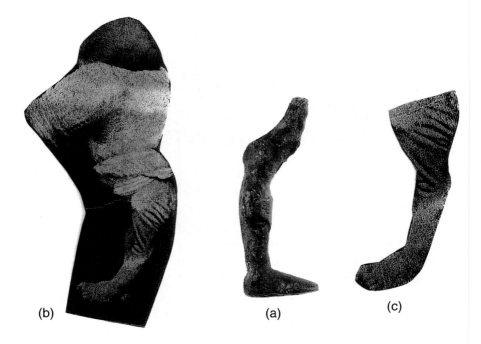

(b)   (a)   (c)

Figure 45
(a) Votive bronze leg (3cm) from the temple of Mercury. This depicts 'back knee' or *genu recurvatum* and dates to between the second and fourth century AD (Photo courtesy Dr Ann Woodward and reproduced with permission from the Trustees of the British Museum © Copyright The British Museum)
(b) Child with *genu recurvatum*. The left leg has been reproduced and (c) the photo enlarged to demonstrate the mirror image depiction by the votive from Uley
(Photocopied from The Doctorate Thesis by Fargeas, JB, Paris 1908 (ref 23, chapter VII))

(dislocation) of the knee joint and may occur as a complication of poliomyelitis, trauma or local inflammatory conditions. Before the days of modern surgical techniques, it was treated by simple immobilization using either splints or bandaging[21,22]. The presence of a votive depicting 'back knee' at a temple of Mercury is compatible with Mercury's role as messenger of the gods: owing to his fleetness of foot, he was credited with the power to treat diseases of the lower extremities [personal communication, Dr M Henig]. This votive may have been given to attract Mercury's attention to the supplicant's affliction or as thanks for treatment of the deformity by rest and immobilization. If the back knee deformity of the votive shown in Figure 45a is not due to purposeful bending at time of donation (as the authors of the report believe), then it is a true depiction of an affliction. This may represent

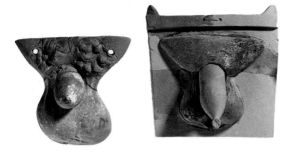

Figure 46 Two of the many votive penises found at Corinth, dating from the late fifth to fourth century BC (Photo © American School of Classical Studies, Corinth Excavations, Athens, Greece)

the earliest evidence for the presence of polio in Roman Britain and, therefore, have major palaeopathological importance.

It is not possible to state that the flaccid penises of Corinth were in fact custom votives (Figure 46). They have been assigned as gifts for treatment of a variety of common genitourinary problems experienced by men; however, when a physician views them, he is tempted to speculate further especially if allowed to present a case study 'cum lingua in bucca', such as the following case report from Corinth:

During a classical Walpurgis nacht[23], a small votive penis was heard to say: 'My master was a very busy man in Rome. He was in the import and export business and he was having trouble with the dock workers at Ostia. He had to spend several hours each week on the crowded roads and would often drink a jug of his own imported wine on the long trip back on the Via Roma. He arrived home at night exhausted and mildly intoxicated. His wife Olivia would berate him for not noticing her new silk gowns and, because of his loss of sexual interest, accused him of seeking diversion in the brothels of the port city. He became unable to perform his manly duties and sought medical help. After trying a variety of treatments including fresh Sylphium from Cyrenaica and rhinoceros horn from India, his doctor sent him to Corinth. The *arch-hetaera* gave him the first treatment and then we had a wonderful time with the others who solicit in the name of Aphrodite. He soon became virile and full of desire and he rushed back to Rome leaving me as a memento of thanks to the Great One.'

The votive tells a true tale. His master suffered from impotency — a condition usually caused by fatigue, debilitation, excess alcohol or psychological stresses. A sojourn at any temple could ameliorate or even eliminate these underlying factors but, in addition, Corinth was noted throughout the Greek and Roman world as a city of licentious libertines. Horace commented that good fortune and great wealth were needed to visit the city and its entertainments. The main temple of Aphrodite was located on the acropolis and crowded with many professional prostitutes (*hetaerae*), whose job was to satisfy supplicants in the name of Aphrodite. There were other temples of Aphrodite at Corinth, some more official than others, but all provided the same basic services.

Sex therapists of today treat impotency by staging a variety of erotic situations; following the first success, the defeatist barrier is broken and replaced by positive thinking and improved performance. The fleshpots of Corinth undoubtedly played a contributing role in the therapeutic success of the Asclepian temple, as did the reassurances received from the extensive display of votives given by cured patients. Perhaps this was why Euripides, the dramatist, chose Corinth as the place for King Aegeus of Athens to seek treatment and help in the conception of his son, Theseus[24]; it may also account for the establishment of an ancillary temple to Aphrodite amid the Asclepian complex at Epidaurus. It is no surprise that archaeology has confirmed Corinth as the urological capital of the ancient world!

Dedications in stone

Votive dedication slabs and votive altars were frequently given to the gods. Inscribed with details about the donor, they resemble modern hospital identification cards used to facilitate correct patient identification. The supplicant wanted to ensure recognition by Asclepius. Dedications in Latin usually ended with the words '*votum solvit libens merito*', frequently shortened to VSLM, which translates as 'willingly and deservedly fulfilled his vow'. However, the donor was sometimes a little more thankful and added '*laetus*' (gladly) to the dedication which then appeared as VSLLM. The deity's name was also abbreviated. Jupiter Optimus Maximus (the best and greatest) became IOM, while Asclepius was often abbreviated to 'ulapio' or 'pio' (Figures 59, 61, 62). Votive dedications were also recorded on metal plaques nailed onto temple walls or thrown into sacred springs and waters[25]. Supplicants sometimes purchased individual letters made from metal with pre-drilled holes for nailing, using them to write their own message. Some of the most notable written testimonials were found at Epidaurus where the priests recorded (for a fee) patients' names and their miraculous cures on stone steles (described in chapter 4).

Votive bas-reliefs donated by wealthy patients are excellent illustrations of Asclepian temple medicine. A tablet found at Thyrea

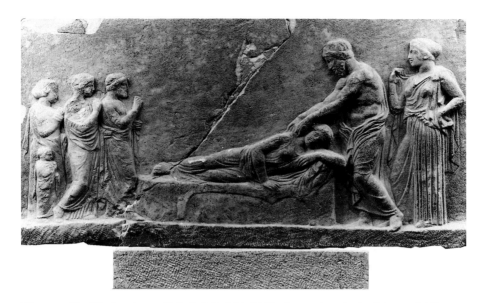

Figure 47 Votive bas-relief (c370–270 BC) from the Asclepieion of Piraeus, depicting Asclepius and Hygieia treating a patient in the company of the patient's family. The sculptor has depicted Hygieia with a prominent goitre (Photo © National Archaeological Museum of Greece, Athens)

in Argolis depicts Asclepius with his sons and daughters towering above six members of a family seeking his help (Figure 15). A relief found in the Asclepieion of Piraeus shows Asclepius and Hygieia treating a patient in the company of the family (Figure 47). The sculptor of this relief carved in excellent detail, depicting Hygieia with a goitre. Thyroid enlargement was common in the mountainous areas of Greece and simple enlargement could not have been considered a symptom of disease otherwise Hygieia would have cured it. Apollo, as well as many other gods, has been portrayed with a goitre (Figure 8c)[26]. A votive relief from the Asclepieion of Athens shows a family sacrificing fruit and cakes to Asclepius and Hygieia[27]; in the background, an obese serpent descends from a tree in anticipation of food. The serpent and tree portrait resembles the depiction on a coin of Caracalla (Figure 21) and the serpent in a bas-relief from Bath (Figure 22).

The Athens National Museum holds a votive tablet from Oropus depicting two female attendants helping a lady to lie down on a bed while the anxious husband hovers in the background[28]. The scene does not depict a woman about to deliver, but it may record the successful end to a difficult delivery with parturition occurring from the sitting position (this tilts the uterus backwards and facilitates delivery).

Chapter 4 mentions briefly the dedications on stone pillars (stelae) found in the *abaton* at Epidaurus. Archaeology revealed the original presence of four stelae with 69 preserved inscriptions dating to the latter part of the fourth century BC when the sanctuary was undergoing reconstruction and expansion. Many classicists have studied their varied messages. Recently, LiDonnici reviewed their context and concluded that the inscriptions were a written abstract describing selected testimonies and votives. These had become superfluous at the time of temple renovation and were due for burial[29]. They expressed the appreciation of supplicants for the incubation ritual fulfilling various requests and their reading would have reassured those who were waiting their turn in the *abaton*. The stelae at Epidaurus are a unique example of an ancient work on medical archives and their earliest inscriptions even record the early association of Apollo with Asclepius.

The Roman empire minted commemorative votive bronze coins every five to 10 years on the occasion of public prayers for the health of the emperor[30]. One such coin showing detailed reference to the myth of Asclepius was described in Chapter 1 (Figure 7).

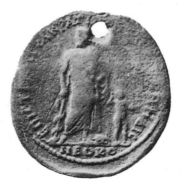

Figure 48 A pierced coin (161–9 AD) from Pergamum depicting Asclepius holding a serpent-entwined staff in his right hand. On his left side there is a small, naked figure with his outstretched left hand, possibly holding a bird. Between them and at their feet, there is a rat gnawing at an unidentified object. The coin is perforated for suspending around the neck (Photo BMC, M&W)

Talismans

A talisman is a charm engraved with a magical symbol believed to have the power to ward off evil and bring about good. Most people in the ancient world held this super-stitious belief. The followers of Asclepius used talismans either to preserve health or to prevent recurrence of an illness; these depicted Asclepius with his serpent, sometimes including Hygieia and Telesphorus. Coins with a portrait of Asclepius were the most con-venient and economical talisman and might be perforated for sus-pension from a necklace or a bracelet (Figure 48). The wealthy wore rings, brooches and pendants made from jewels into which the magic symbol had been cut in cameo or intaglio format. Dr Henig

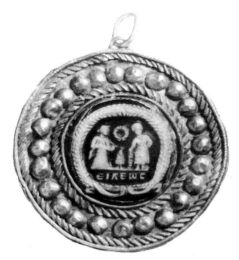

Figure 49 Gold pendant of the third century AD showing Asclepius, Hygieia and Telesphorus and inscribed 'ειλεως' (ileus) (Photo by Robert Wilkins FSA and reproduced courtesy Dr Martin Henig, Institute of Archaeology, Oxford, England and the Content Family Collection of Ancient Cameos, Houlton, Maine, US)

of the Institute of Archaeology at Oxford described a unique example of an Asclepian talisman that was set in a handsome gold pendant of third century design. This depicts Asclepius holding his serpent-entwined staff and wearing a Phrygian cap, and he is accompanied by Hygieia holding a serpent and Telesphorus standing between them. Beneath this medical trinity is the inscription ειλεως (eileos) which translates to 'ileus' or paralytic bowel obstruction (Figure 49)[31,32]. The pendant was found in Syria and the Phrygian cap suggests that it is the Phoenician Eshmun-Asclepius who is depicted. The addition of Telesphorus and Hygieia indicates a return to health after a period of convalescence.

An intaglio ring, depicting Asclepius and Hygieia and engraved with the Greek letters APE (possibly short for *arete*), the Greek word for virtue, was found at Braintree, Essex, England[33]. This ring may have belonged to either a doctor or patient, but it is unclear why it was found at this rural location in Roman Britain. Stane Street, one of the main Roman roads running west from the nearby Roman town of Camulodunum (Colchester), runs through present-day Braintree. Colchester was the first major town in Roman Britain with *Colonia* status, a temple of Claudius and a mint. Four Roman oculist's stamps (the largest number from a single site in Britain)[6] and several surgical instruments including a complete basic surgical kit have been found there. These probably belonged to physicians associated with the Roman army who may have set up a civilian practice after their discharge from military service. The physicians would have worshipped Aesculapius and one wonders whether or not they had a shrine to Aesculapius that their patients could visit. The proximity of Braintree to Colchester is an adequate explanation for the presence of this talisman dedicated to Asclepius. An intaglio of Hygieia wearing a *himation* and feeding a serpent coiled around a tree was found in the area of *praetentura* of the Roman fort at Brecon, Wales[34]. This may have belonged to the physician associated with the fort and its discovery provides the most westerly evidence for Asclepius in the Roman empire.

Notes and references

1. Jackson R. *Doctors and diseases in the Roman empire*. London: British Museum Press, 1988.
2. Lang M. *Cure and cult in ancient Corinth. American excavations in old Corinth. Corinth notes no 1*. Athens: American School of Classical Studies of Athens, 1977.
3. Barker PA, White RH, Pretty KB *et al. Excavation of the site of the Baths and Basilica, Wroxeter 1966–1990*. London: English Heritage.
4. Wright T. *Uriconium: an account of the ancient Roman city at Wroxeter*. London: Private Printing, 1872.
5. Barnes H. On Roman medicine and Roman medical inscriptions found in Britain. *Proc R Soc Med* 1914; 7 (History of Medicine Section): 71.
6. Jackson R. A new collyrium stamp from Cambridge and a corrected reading of the stamp from Caister-by-Norwich. *Britannia* 1990; **21**: 275–83.
7. Celsus. *De Medicina*. Translated by Spencer WG. Book 6. Massachusetts: Harvard University Press, 1953: 3–6.
8. Woodward A. *Shrines and sacrifice*. London: English Heritage, 1992.
9. Meyer-Steineg T. *Jenaer Medizin-Historische Beitrage*. No 2. Jena, 1912.
10. McCord CD, Spitalny LA. Generalized orbital varices. *Arch Ophthal* 1968; **80**: 455–60.
11. Lloyd CAS, Wright JE, Morgan G. Venous malformations of the orbit. *Br J Ophthalmol* 1971; **55**: 505–16.
12. Orbital varices. [Editorial.] *BMJ* 1971; **4**: 764.
13. Allison-Jones L. *Women in Roman Britain*. London: British Museum Publications, 1989.
14. Wheeler REM, Wheeler TV. *Report of the prehistoric, Roman, and post-Roman site in Lydney Park, Gloucestershire*. London: The Society of Antiquaries, 1932.
15. Hart GD. A hematological artifact from fourth century Britain. *Bull Hist Med* 1970; **44**(1): 76–9.
16. Allison-Jones L. *Women in Roman Britain*. London: British Museum Publications, 1989.
17. This 'old wives tale' was still heard by midwives practising in Britain during the early 1950s.
18. Woodward AB, Leach PJ. *The Uley shrines. Excavation of a ritual complex on West Hill, Uley, Gloucestershire, 1977–9*. London: English Heritage in association with British Museum Press, 1993.

19. Hopperfield S. *Physical examination of the spine and extremities*. Connecticut: Appleton-Century-Crofts, 1976: 172

20. Ingram AJ. *Genu recurvatum*. In: Crenshaw AH, ed. *Operative orthopaedics*. Toronto: The CV Mosby Company, 1987.

21. Keen WW. *Surgery: its principles and practice*. *Volume 2*. Philadelphia: WB Saunders Company, 1908: 539–40, 581.

22. Fargeas JB. *Étude sur l'absence congénitale de la rotule. Thèse pour Le Doctoriat en Médecine*. Paris: Jouve et Boyer, 1908.

23. The eve of May Day was an occasion for high revelry in the witch world; festivities were celebrated on the highest point of the Harz Mountains. Walpurgis was an English nun who went to Germany as a missionary and became the abbess of Heidenheim. Her day is 1st May, hence her association with the earlier pagan festival. Goethe, in *Faust* Part II, described a classical Walpurgis nacht where all the spirits of the classical world assembled and celebrated.

24. Euripides, *The Medea*, translated by Rex Warner. Chicago: The University of Chicago Press, 1955.

25. Many of the inscriptions on metal plaques contained complaints, curses and problems of a personal nature.

26. Hart GD. Even the gods had goitre. *Can Med Assoc J* 1967; **96**: 1432–6.

27. This is illustrated in: Kerenyi C. *Asklepios*. New York: Pantheon Books Inc, 1959: 33.

28. An illustration of this appears in: Margotta R. *An illustrated history of medicine*. Middlesex: Hamlyn Publishing Group, 1968: 59.

29. LiDonnici LR. Compositional background of the Epidaurian Iamata. *Am J Philology* 1992; **113**: 26–41.

30. Gerlitt J. Votive offerings. *Ciba Symposia* 1939; **1**: no 4.

31. Henig M. An inscribed intaglio. *Britannia* 1983; **16**: 241–2.

32. Dr Henig's colleague, Mr Dimitris Plantzos, feels the inscription could be a form of address to the gods meaning propitious.

33. Henig M. Inscribed intaglio. *Britannia* 1985; **16**: 241–2.

34. Henig M. *A corpus of Roman engraved gemstones from British sites*. 2nd edn. BAR British Series 8. 1978: 285.

Chapter 7

Rome adopts Asclepius

Asclepius arrives in Rome

In 293 BC, Rome was ravaged by an uncontrolled epidemic and civic authorities were obliged to seek the assistance of a Greek deity. Many ancient authors have described the events leading to the adoption of Asclepius into the Roman pantheon and the subsequent restoration of health to 'the capital of the world'[1]:

> 'Once upon a time there was a lethal plague that had infected the air of Latium: human bodies lay wasting away and ashen-faced with debilitating sickness. People realised that all their human efforts were to no avail and that the skill of the healer could achieve nothing; and so they sought divine assistance.' Ovid, *Metamorphoses* XV, 626–30 (ET 850)

The Senate responded to the growing emergency and consulted the Sibylline Books:

> 'In the Books they found that it was necessary to summon Asclepius to Rome from Epidaurus; but they could do nothing about it that year, because the consuls were busy waging war.' Livy, *Ab Urbe Condita*, X, 47,7 (ET 583)

Some senators were reluctant to accept this advice, which recommended replacement of their Apollo Medicus by an unknown, foreign deity. Seeking a second opinion, they went to the temple of Apollo at Delphi where they consulted his oracle. This was their reply:

> 'You do not need Apollo to soothe your troubles but Apollo's son. Go with favourable omens and seek my son's assistance.' Ovid, *Metamorphoses* XV, 638–40 (ET 850)[2]

Due to either the war or political inertia, the Senate continued to postpone seeking Aesculapius' help. Eventually, in 291 BC, they were prepared to sponsor the religious preparations required for adopting a powerful, foreign god into their own pantheon. Quintus Ogulnius was appointed to lead a delegation of 10 senators to Epidaurus. They received an ambivalent reception from some of the city elders who were reluctant to allow their own source of wealth to leave the city. Ovid reported that the god himself resolved the problem by speaking first to the Roman diplomat in a dream and then to the councillors of Epidaurus:

'Do not be afraid! I will come and I will leave my shrine. Just look at this serpent which is entwined about my staff; make a careful note so that you may recognise it. I shall change myself into this, but I will be larger and will seem the same size as the heavenly bodies are when they change.' Ovid, *Metamorphoses* XV, 658–62 (ET 850)

The Epidaurian elders assembled in the temple of Asclepius, at the foot of his gold and ivory statue (Figure 6), and begged him to solve their dilemma:

'They had scarcely stopped speaking when the golden god, in the form of a serpent with his crest held high, made hissing noises warning of his presence. As he came, the statue, the altars, the doors, the marble floor and the gilded roof all shook. Then he stood there chest-high in the middle of the temple gazing around, his eyes flashing with fire. The terrified crowd trembled with fright; but the priest whose sacred locks were tied with a white fillet recognised the god and cried: "It's the God! Look it's the God! Think holy thoughts and stand in silent reverence, all you who stand in his presence. And, you, most beautiful one, may your appearance before us bring us good fortune and may you bless your people who worship you at your temple!" ... The god nodded approvingly to them and, motioning with his crest, assured them of his favour and with tongue quivering, he continued to hiss repeatedly. Then he slid down the polished steps and looking backwards with eyes fixed on the ancient altars he was about to leave, bade farewell to the home he knew so well and to the temple where he had lived so long.' Ovid, *Metamorphoses* XV, 669–87[1,3]

The narrative then described Asclepius' passage through the city to the boat and the details of his voyage to Rome. The vessel stopped at Antium, due to either rough waters or on Asclepius' request, where he disembarked and visited the temple of Apollo[4]. He stayed there for three days, coiled around branches of a palm tree in the outer courtyard of the temple. This sojourn would have been useful for messengers to notify Rome of the expected arrival time, to allow for preparations of an appropriate welcome for the 'Saviour of the City'. The ship then sailed north to the mouth of the River Tiber. Ovid described Asclepius' triumphal entry into Rome:

'Out came the whole mass of the population to meet him from every direction: mothers and fathers and the virgins who look after your fire, O Trojan Vesta, greeted the god with their cheering. And where the speedy ship came floating up stream, incense crackled and burned on altars erected at regular intervals along both banks and the air was heavy with fragrance. The sacrificial beast, as it was hit, warmed the priest's knife with blood. Now the ship entered Rome, the capital of the world. The serpent raised himself up and, placing his head upon the top mast, he moved it from side to side, looking out for somewhere suitable to live. The river, as it flows along, divides at this point into two streams, forming a place known as "the island"; on both sides it stretches out two equal arms with the land in between. This is the place where the serpent- son of Phoebus Apollo came out from the Latin ship and, turning back into his heavenly form, brought the people's woes to an end and came to them as bringer of health to their city.' Ovid, *Metamorphoses* XV, 729–44[5]

Some authors state that Asclepius jumped out of the boat and swam to the island: '... and when the ambassadors had got out of the boat onto the bank of the Tiber, he swam over to the island, where a temple has been erected in his honour.' Valerius Maximus (ET 848)

Asclepius' arrival at the island in the Tiber was commemorated on a votive medallion struck by Antoninus Pius in 140–3 AD (Figure 50). The centre of this beautiful bronze engraving depicts Asclepius in the form of a huge serpent, with his head and body thrusting forward from the prow of the ship; below him is Faunus, god of the island's sacred spring, welcoming Asclepius with an offering of a river bird. The ship, a galley with rowers, has a river pilot or captain standing on the foredeck as it passes under the arches of the Pons Aemilius[6]. The tower, pediment and entablature depicted on the island was a conjectural representation of the island skyline in the third century BC.

The arrival of Asclepius in Rome was also commemorated on a coin minted in 83 BC by Senator Lucius Rubrius Dossenus, descendant of an original emissary to Epidaurus. This coin depicts a bistyle temple with a large serpent rearing from the altar and a ship's prow in the background[7] (Figure 51). It probably shows Asclepius in his temple at

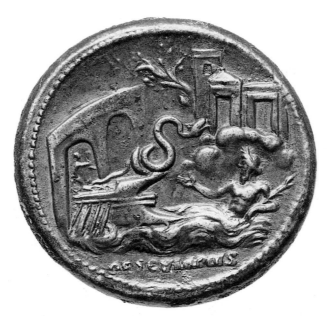

Figure 50 Medallion commemorating the arrival of Asclepius in Rome and the establishment of his temple on the island in the Tiber (Photo © Bibliothèque Nationale de France, Service Photographique, Paris, France)

Epidaurus. The boat was the vessel carrying Dossenus' ancestor to Epidaurus and that brought Asclepius to Rome. Dossenus also minted a coin portraying a snake-entwined altar or possibly the well head of the temple of Aesculapius at Rome. Both coins may have been minted to propitiate Aesculapius and beseech his help to end the epidemic following the social war and the siege of Rome. There is a discrepancy

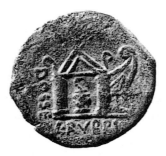

Figure 51 Bronze coin commemorating Senator Dossenus' ancestor who went to Epidaurus to bring Asclepius to Rome (Photo © Bibliothèque Nationale de France, Service Photographique, Paris, France)

in the assigned date for these coins — Roquefeuil states 83 BC and Foss c87 BC[7].

Island in the Tiber

The island in the Tiber is located in the heart of Rome; its ancient name of Insula Tiberina is still used and is called the Isola in modern Italian. Legend ascribed the formation of the island to the Etruscan ruler, Tarquin the Proud, and his followers throwing wheat into the river at the time of their expulsion from Rome:

> 'And there exists even at the present time a prominent reminder of this event that once took place, namely, the large island sacred to Aesculapius, which is washed all round by the river...' Dionysius of Halicarnassus, *Antiquitates Romanae,* Vol 13, 4 (ET 857)

Whatever the truth about its origin, the island is considered to have been a sacred place. Its choice for the site of the temple of Aesculapius followed the tradition of continuity of sanctity whereby people of different cultures and religious beliefs built their shrines on sites used in earlier times[8,9]. Part of a terracotta antefix, thought to be from the wall of a religious building, was found some years ago. It was considered too early in date to be associated with the third century temple of Aesculapius. Further evidence of the antiquity of worship on the island is suggested by its association with an early Latin underground deity named Vediovis, often associated with Jupiter and to whom a temple was erected in 194 BC. It was Vediovis who sent the plague and its cure, and who later became the god of asylum and protector of slaves. Then there was Semo Sancus (Dius Fidius), a native Italian cult figure associated with the Sabine people. An inscription of the second century date refers to a statue dedicated to this god. There was also the rural god Faunus, god of forests and protector of flocks, who was venerated on the island. In 196 BC, a temple to Faunus was built with money collected in the form of fines from fraudsters. The burial grounds of the Campus Martius were on the opposite bank of the river and the nearby flour mills of the Tiber were associated with the goddess Ceres. Fortuitously, the island was located upstream from the *cloaca maxima* (main sewer of Rome) and distant from the malarial-infested marshes draining into the Tiber[10]. If Vitruvius had been available for consultation in 291 BC, he too would have selected the Island!

January 1, the most holy date in the Roman calendar, was chosen to be the day to dedicate the founding of the temple of Asclepius.

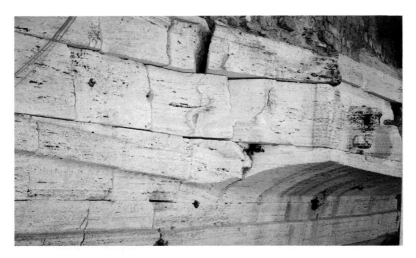

Figure 52 The preserved boat-shaped prow of the third century BC Aesculapian temple at Rome. The rope above is coincidental but could well be a mooring line! (Photo GDH)

'... it was on this day that the senate dedicated two temples. The island, enclosed by the river's divided water, became the home to the one whom the nymph Coronis bore to Phoebus Apollo. Jupiter also shares the place. A single site made room for both of them and the temple of the almighty grandfather and grandson are coupled together.' Ovid, *Fasti*, I, 290–94 (ET 855)

Archaeology and legend

The island's temple of Aesculapius had a unique design commemorating his dramatic entry into Rome. The island itself was converted into the shape of a ship's hull, its sides constructed of travertine marble with contours preventing the swiftly flowing waters of the Tiber from eroding the temple complex foundations. The boat-like platform was constructed with the bow facing downstream (west) and the stern resisting the current (east)[11]. After 23 centuries, in spite of the destruction caused by time, wars and religious zealots, a large fragment of the port side prow of the ship still rises 10 feet above the level of its ancient dock. The carved blocks of marble have retained their graceful shape and still curve downwards to form the keel, outwards to shape the hull and inwards to converge on the point of the prow (Figure 52). Carved in the area on the bow where vessels display their name, there is a serpent-entwined staff and a time-eroded bust of Aesculapius who peers in ghostly fashion over the ruins of the ancient city, totally oblivious to the roar of motor traffic on the 'left' bank (Figure 53).

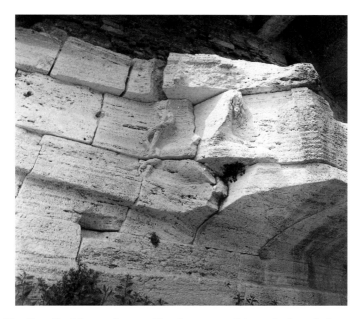

Figure 53   Detail of the ancient staff and serpent of Aesculapius, dating to the third century BC, still preserved on the bank of the island in the Tiber (Photograph courtesy of the Photographic Department Ospedale Fatebenefratelli, Isola, Rome, Italy)

Here, archaeology unites the mythology of the past with the reality of the present.

In the third century AD, the temple complex was divided into two sections by an obelisk, creating the illusion of a ship's mast[12]. The temple proper and its healing spring were sited at the western end of the island under the present church of San Bartolomeo, and the other temple buildings were located under the present Ospedale dei Fatebenefratelli (see chapter 11). Several pits containing votives have been excavated on the island and a statue of Aesculapius has been retrieved from the river. The spring is presently capped but the well head is still in situ. An esplanade has been added around the original buildings and an aerial view of the island resembles a modern ocean liner rather than a Roman galley[13] (Plan 5). Jumbled blocks of stone in the river around the periphery of the island, undoubtedly derived from the temple complex, provide teasing pieces of archaeological jigsaw.

Four votive testimonies to Aesculapius on the island were recorded in *Inscriptiones Graecae* XIV, 966 (ET 438); three of these are quoted below:

'To Lucius, who was sick with pleurisy and had been despaired of by everyone, the god advised that he should go and gather ashes from

Plan 5   Island in the Tiber (Insula)

C Buhle

1. Tiber with direction of flow
2. Insula
3. Present-day hospital (Ospedale Fatebenefratelli)
4. Modern pharmacy
5. Courtyard with fountain
6. Modern stairway surrounded by temple walls
7. Corridor with glass floor leading to diagnostic
   imaging department with temple walls visible below
8. Pons Fabricius built 62 BC (Ponte dei Quattro Capi)
   which links the island to the left bank
9. Statues depicting a duplicate head of
   Janus
10. Pons Cestius built 46 BC (Ponte San Bartolomeo)
    joins the island to the right bank (Trastevere)
11. Pons Aemilius built 179 BC was depicted on the
    medallion of Antoninus Pius (Figure 57). The bridge
    is now a ruin and named Ponte Rotto

12. Ponte Palatino which carries modern
    traffic from the north side of the Tiber
    towards the Circus Maximus, the
    Colosseum and the Forum
13. *Cloaca maxima* — the principal sewer
    of ancient Rome
14. Church of San Bartolomeo built over
    the site of the temple of Aesculapius
15. Site of the healing spring of the temple
    of Aesculapius. The same waters were
    also used in Christian healing
16. Remains of the prow of the ship-shaped
    temple of Aesculapius and the site of the
    staff of Aesculapius
17. Site of the earliest Jewish hospital in
    Rome

the threefold altar and that he should mix them well with wine and put them on the side of his chest. And he was saved and gave thanks to the god in public.'

'To Julian, who was spitting up blood and had been despaired of by everyone, the god advised that he should go and take the seed of a pine cone from the threefold altar and he should eat them together with some honey for three days. And he was saved . . .'

'To Valerius Aper, a blind soldier, the god advised that he should go and take the blood of a white cock along together with some honey and that he should concoct an eye salve and that he should apply it for three days . . .'

These testimonies indicate that the temple had a threefold altar, the ashes and wine acted as an ancient 'mustard plaster' for treating pleurisy, and that a mixture of pine cones and honey was prescribed as a cough expectorant and suppressant. In addition to its focus on healing and health, the island acquired another function on January 1 194 BC when a temple was dedicated to Vediovis. Two and a half centuries later, we learn that Emperor Claudius, who famously placed great trust in former slaves as his aids, acted generously towards slaves who had been abandoned on Tiber island:

'When some people were exposing their sick and exhausted slaves on the island of Aesculapius because they could not be bothered to treat them, he [Claudius] decreed that all those that had been exposed should be freed: if they recovered, they should not return to the jurisdiction of their master. But if anyone preferred to kill such a slave rather than expose him he should be charged with murder.' Suetonius, *Claudius*, 25, 2 (ET 858)

Island bridges
The island has a special relationship with the ancient bridges of Rome. The earliest bridge across the Tiber was the wooden Pons Sublicius, built by Etruscan carpenters in around the sixth century BC. At this bridge, which lies a little further down the river, Horatius, Herminius and Spurius Lartius stalled the attacking Etruscans when they tried to re-enter the city. Aesculapius sailed under this bridge when he entered Rome in 291 BC.

Pons Aemilius, constructed by Aemilius Lepidus in 179 BC, is the bridge depicted on the medallion of Antoninus Pius (Figure 50). This

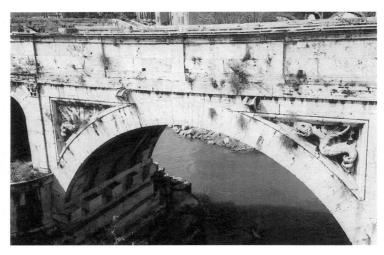

Figure 54   Modern view of the ancient (179 BC) arch of the Ponto Rotto with the tip of the island showing. This would have been the first view of the island in the story as told by Ovid (Photo GDH)

was the first bridge over the Tiber to be built on stone piers; it continued to carry traffic from the north side of the Tiber to the Colosseum and the Circus Maximus until 1598 AD, when all but one arch collapsed. The remaining central arch, decorated with ornate Roman and Papal bas-reliefs, has, along with its now-isolated roadway, been re-named Ponte Rotto (Broken Bridge) (Figure 54).

The pedestrian and road traffic to and from the island would have caused traffic gridlock in the capital of the ancient world. This problem was resolved by building two additional bridges, Pons Cestius and Pons Fabricius, that connected the island to both shores of the Tiber. Pons Cestius, built in 46 BC, continues to carry pedestrians between the island and the right bank (Trastevere). It has acquired a new name, Ponte San Bartolomeo, as well as the 20th century burden of Vespas, Fiats and Ferraris. The original arches of Pons Fabricius, constructed in the time of Cicero (62 BC), continue to span the Tiber and carry pedestrian traffic from the left bank. Two Janus heads guard each side of the mainland entrance to the bridge.

Janus was a Roman solar deity distinct from any of the Greek gods. As the god of departures and returns, he had two faces so he could observe those entering and leaving all doorways. As god of beginnings, he was associated with the start of the new year—the month January derives from his name; the first day of each month was also dedicated to him. Janus was an extremely important god to the Romans and was referred to as the 'god of gods'. He was depicted on the earliest Roman

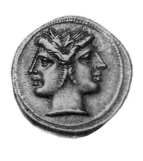

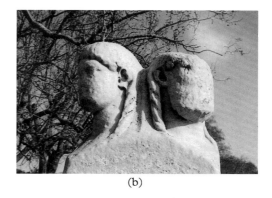

(a)   (b)

Figure 55
(a) Silver didrachm of Rome (c215–212 BC) showing a beardless Janus (Photo CNG)
(b) The four heads, dating to 62 BC, still guarding the entrance to the Ponte dei
Quattro Capi (Photo GDH)

coins both with and without a beard (Figure 55a). The unusual
depictions at the entrance to the Pons Fabricius is explained by the
double dedications on the day of Janus, one to the temple to Jupiter-
Aesculapius and the other to Vediovis. The Janus of Aesculapius and
Vediovis were combined with the result that the entrance is guarded in
four directions; the modern name of the bridge is, thus, Ponte dei
Quattro Capi — Bridge of Four Heads (Figure 55b).

Aesculapius elsewhere in Rome

Another sanctuary of Aesculapius was located in the *Regia Pontificis*,
the official residence of the *Pontifex Maximus* (chief priest of Roman
religion)[14]. This shrine communicated with a medicinal pool separate
from the pool of the Regia; it is tempting to speculate that the former
was reserved for high officialdom. Other statues to Aesculapius stood
nearby in the forum, one in the atrium of the Vestal Virgins and
another in the temple of Concord (ET 661). There was also a famous
statue sculptured by Cephisodotus, the son of Praxiteles, in the
colonnade of Octavia in the temple of Juno (ET 651). Augustus
rewarded his personal physician, Antonius Musa, with a sculpture
depicting Musa as Aesculapius (ET 644). This was erected beside an
existing statue of Aesculapius and symbolized the father–son
relationship of the Asclepiads to Aesculapius.

Rome and the Asclepiads

Even after adopting Aesculapius into the Roman pantheon, the city
distrusted Greek physicians. Senator Cato (234–149 BC), a noted
critic of the increasing influence of Hellenic culture in Rome, was one

of their most outspoken opponents and voiced the opinion that they constituted a threat to Roman health. Pliny recorded that he wrote the following to his son:

> 'If that pack pass onto us what they know, it will mean the end of Rome, especially if their doctors come here. For they have sworn death by medicine to the barbarians and the Roman are barbarians to them. Beware of doctors!'[15]

For this reason, early Greek doctors in the city did not wish to emphasize their Greek origins and were happy to use the Latin name *medicus* than convert the epithet Asclepiad into a Latin format.

Archagathus of Sparta, who established a practice at the Acilian crossroads (219 BC), has been credited as the first Greek doctor with a civic appointment in Rome[16]. In 58 BC, the moneyer Manius Acilius Glabrio minted a coin depicting the goddesses Salus and Valetudo that proudly proclaimed 'the legend' that a member of his family had introduced the first Greek physician to Rome (Figure 56). Salus had a double role in the Roman world; not only was she associated with health, she also symbolized the safety of the state as well as the health and restorative power of the emperor. Salus' depiction on the obverse was symbolic of her civic role while Valetudo with a serpent, on the reverse, was a symbol of her medical role. The 'VIR III' inscription represented 'the board of [three] magistrates who controlled the mint'. This coin is of great significance as it indicates that, by this date, Greek physicians had been accepted by Roman society.

Rome appeared to experience a shortage of doctors because many emperors offered inducements for new practitioners. In 46 BC, Julius

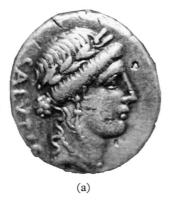
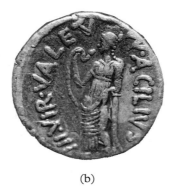

(a)   (b)

Figure 56 Silver denarius which depicted (a) the laureate head of Salus on the obverse and (b) Valetudo on the reverse (Photo GDH)

Caesar granted citizenship to all foreign doctors practising in Rome; unfortunately, there was no method of licensing at that time and followers of other medical doctrines, as well as charlatans and quacks, benefited from his decree[17]. In 10 AD, Augustus granted physicians exemption from taxes and Vespasian introduced a form of socialized medicine that recruited doctors to become civic employees (*circulatores*), responsible for visiting outlying areas and treating those unable to afford medical care. Such physicians, who were also exempt from paying tax and compulsory service, were given 'clinic facilities'. Communities also appointed a chief physician (*archiatrus*) who enjoyed a variety of desirable privileges including magisterial powers and, on occasion, the responsibility for minting coins on which he inscribed his name and the title *archiatros*[18]. Appointments for civic physicians became so popular that, in 160 AD, Emperor Antoninus Pius placed a limit on the number of positions available and restricted civic budgets to 10 physicians in capital cities, seven in large towns and five in small towns[19]. In spite of Roman awareness of public health and the need for a crowded urban population, qualifications of early physicians were poorly documented. The Romans did not have a background of legislation for qualifying doctors until the third century when Severus Alexander (222–35 AD) passed laws regulating the training, certification and licensing of doctors.

Aesculapius castrorum

Roman army camps maintained scrupulous hygienic conditions by means of ensuring a supply of pure water, elaborate drains, latrines and bathing facilities. In addition to these measures for maintaining health among their soldiers, the army attracted or conscripted Greek doctors into its ranks. These *medici* travelled with the troops and spread their worship of Aesculapius throughout the Roman empire to such a degree that Aesculapius acquired the epithet 'Aesculapius castrorum'— Asclepius of the camps.

The medical needs of the army were divided between those required for battle conditions and those in camp life both behind the lines and at times of peace. The military seized the opportunity to enlist the skills of the Greek physicians. Each doctor who joined the army took the military oath and became a soldier (*miles*), although his duties did not necessarily involve fighting and certain other military activities; this special status was indicated by the title of '*miles immunis*'. The title '*miles medicus*' possibly designated a doctor who had received on the job training while serving in the ranks; training under these circumstances for removing embedded missiles may have been superior to that of the

Greek doctors! Perhaps some of these doctors were the average rank and were file army recruits who had learnt their skill on the job and acquired the title '*medicus ordinarius*'[20,21].

The *milites medici* resemble today's doctors who join the army for a career. They assessed the soldier's fitness to serve, became camp doctors and treated the 'sick' who suffered from infectious diseases, nutritional deficiencies, psychological disorders and other medical problems needing less degree of skill than that of the surgeon. After completing their term of duty (thought to be around 25 years), they were discharged with citizenship, a pension and a land grant that usually occurred at their local region of duty[22]. It was here where many physicians set up civilian practice and indirectly helped to romanize the native populations.

Treating battle injuries required a skilled surgeon; some physicians joined the army to increase their surgical skills. Surgeons were not stationed in the battlefield but were located at the camp hospital (*valetudinarium*) where better facilities for major surgical procedures were available. Emergency treatment in the field was given by the medical orderlies (*capsularii*), named after the bandage box (*capsa*) they carried. These medical orderlies were skilled in emergency treatment and their role was depicted on Trajan's Column in Rome, showing them in ordinary soldier's dress attending the wounded on the battlefield.

The *valetudinaria* were built to a standardized plan, but the dimensions of the building varied in proportion to the number of men stationed there or to the number of soldiers of the vicinity liable to battle injury. They were located behind the camp headquarters building, which was usually the quietest part of the fort. The building was rectangular in shape and had a rectangular inner corridor separating ranges of rooms on each side. The inner rooms faced onto a quadrangle and were possibly occupied by convalescents who would have easy access to the quad for exercise and solar therapy without disturbing other patients. The area was also used for growing medicinal herbs and green vegetables; convalescent soldiers would be ideal 'volunteers' to assist in their cultivation (cultivating vegetables would be good rehabilitation for cutting a vallum!).

The corridor, illuminated by clerestory windows, did not form an integral part of the ward structure but was joined to it at regular intervals by a roofed passageway. The large hall at the entrance served as a triage area at times of heavy casualties. Individual rooms on a ward measured approximately 13 feet by 14 feet (4 metres by 4.25 metres) and accommodated two to eight beds; by serendipity, the layout of the partitions and entrances helped minimize cross infections. There were operating room facilities and a separate kitchen and latrines, as well as medical and administrative space.

The legionary hospitals were extensive and the largest one found to date was located at Vetera on the Rhine (present-day Xanten) which occupied an area of 6,890 square metres; a complete legionary hospital has been identified at Inchtuthill (Perthshire, Scotland) which occupied an area of 5,351 square metres. However, the building was never used and was dismantled when Rome abandoned its plan to conquer all of Caledonia (Scotland)[23,24]. Many of the smaller forts also had hospitals of a proportionately smaller size. Several of these have been found in Roman Britain, the best of which to visit is on Hadrian's Wall at Housesteads (Vercovicium) where the tombstone of a *medicus ordinarius*, who died at 25 years of age, was found[25].

The camp prefect, who had the title '*optio valetudinarii*', controlled the hospital and other camp buildings. The medical officer in charge was the '*medicus castrorum*' or '*medicus castrensis*' who was also responsible for the *medici* and *capsularii*.

Physicians with higher ranks probably had a separate term of duty and, perhaps, served 'on contract.' Some, like Dioscorides and Scribonius Largus, joined the army to take advantage of the opportunity to study plants and herbs with medicinal properties, as well as disease and health problems in distant lands. These special physicians may have helped the army avoid massive casualties of disease, such as that which occurred during the Parthian Campaign when Marcus Antonius (Mark Antony) lost more than one-half of his troops from infection. Good vision was a prime requirement for army recruits and eye diseases were a serious problem among soldiers in foreign lands. It is likely that camp doctors were able to treat eye infections but there may have been a regional 'consultant' (*medicus ocularis*) who not only knew about eye diseases but also acted as quartermaster for the supplies of various eye ointments (*collyria*). One such consultant was Axius ophthalmicus of the British Fleet, who was described by Galen as the originator of the salve of Axius[26].

The *medicus castrorum* or a legion (*medicus legionis*) attained equestrian rank; their military service gained them political and social friends who served them well in civilian practice after discharge from the army. Their educational background facilitated friendships with aristocratic senior officers deprived of intellectual stimulation while on duty with their legions at isolated outposts. The Praetorian Guard, as the emperor's bodyguard, was the most prestigious unit in the Roman army; its first cohort had a *medicus chirugicus* (surgeon) and a *medicus clinicus* (physician). It is likely that this format was the role model for ideal military medical care and the division of medical duties between surgeon and physician was adapted and modified for use with the legions in the field. For the legate or provincial governors, there were also private physicians who served without rank as they were part of a retinue or were hired on a private basis.

The knowledge of military medical organization is better known than its civilian counterpart. However, many gaps still remain in our present-day understanding of the exact structure of the Roman army medical service, and readers are referred to the works of experts in this field[20,21,27] and later studies as they are published.

Aesculapius goes to Britain

The first Asclepiad in the Roman army to gain great fame was Stertinius Xenophon, who became personal physician to Emperor Claudius. He accompanied Claudius on the successful invasion of Britain in 43 AD and was responsible for the medical arrangements of the 40,000–50,000 soldiers in the invading army. After the victory, he was rewarded with the titles 'chief doctor of the divine emperors', 'secretary in charge of Greek affairs', 'military tribune' and 'engineer'; he was also honoured with a gold crown and spear at Rome during Claudius' British triumph (Figure 57)[28]. Some historians have not understood the significance of his title of secretary for Greek affairs and his military rank. These were not token appointments as a Roman military force of this size needed 50–70 physicians, most of whom were probably Greek-trained who needed supplies from their homeland and assistance with communication. The legions established in Britain were stationed in legionary fortresses built along standard lines; each probably had a hospital capable of accommodating 200–300 patients. Xenophon's title of engineer (*praefectus fabrum*) may have referred to hospital construction which conformed to a basic fortress plan similar to that uncovered at Vetera (Germany) and Inchtuthill (Scotland)[23,24].

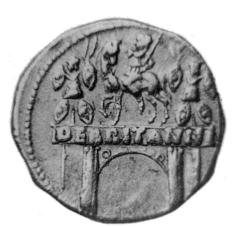

Figure 57 Gold coin of Claudius depicting his Victory Arch erected in Rome in 44 AD to commemorate his successful invasion of south-eastern Britain (Photo CNG, 1993, Vol XVIII, 3)

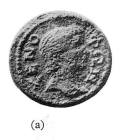
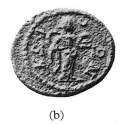
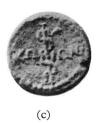

(a)   (b)   (c)

Figure 58
(a) The obverse of a coin of Cos from the second century AD which depicts the famous Coan Asclepiad Xenophon whose association with Emperor Claudius brought honour to the island
(b) The reverse depicts Hygieia holding a large serpent
(c) A similar but smaller coin also depicting Xenophon exists but this shows the staff of Aesculapius on its reverse. This smaller coin is the same size and has the same reverse as the coin in Figure 20 depicting Hippocrates. This pair of coins links the fame of Xenophon to that of Hippocrates
(Photo BMC, M&W)

Having gained great favour with Claudius, Xenophon was able to obtain privileges for his native island of Cos; these included amnesty from paying tribute and the re-establishment of the right of sanctuary. The Coans recorded his fame and memory posthumously by dedicating a small temple to him at their Asclepieion; in the second century AD, they minted a coin which depicted his profile on the obverse and the staff of Aesculapius on the reverse (Figure 58).

Scribonius Largus, who also accompanied Claudius on his invasion of Britain, gained fame from his study of pharmacy. His texts, *De compositione medicamentorum*, were dedicated to Claudius and became the standard pharmacopoeia of the first century (chapter 8).

Greek doctors in the Roman army introduced Aesculapius to the troops who gave him the epithet 'Aesculapius castrorum'. They spread Graeco-Roman medicine and Aesculapian worship into the northern and western parts of the Roman empire, where altars and dedications to Aesculapius were erected. The military's faith in Aesculapius and Salus is reflected by the altar dedicated to him and by the household staff of the imperial legate of the second legion stationed at Chester (Deva), England. One side of this altar depicts his serpent-entwined staff (Figures 59). Also at Chester, when it was the home of the 20th legion (Valeria Victrix), a Greek inscription on an altar reads: 'The doctor Antiochus honours the all-surpassing saviour of men among the immortals, Asclepius of the gentle hands, Hygieia and Panacea.' (Figure 60)[29].

(a)

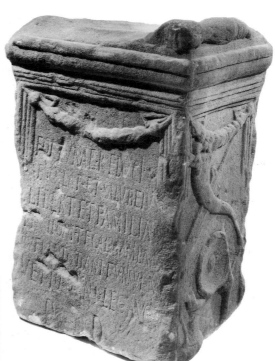

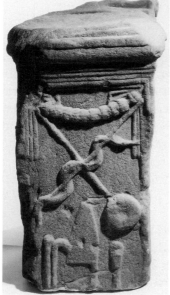

(b)

Figure 59
(a) Altar (50 cm×72.5 cm RIB 445) dedicated to Aesculapius and Salus by the household staff of the imperial legate of the Legion at Deva (Chester) inscribed: 'To fortune the home-bringer, to Aesculapius and to Salus the freedmen and the slave household of TITUS...of the Galerian voting-tribe, imperial legate, gave and dedicated this.' It probably dates to the first half of the second century AD (Photo © Copyright The British Museum)
(b) Staff of Aesculapius, accompanied by sacrificial instruments depicted on the side of the altar (photo © Copyright The British Museum and reproduced courtesy of the Trustees of the British Museum)

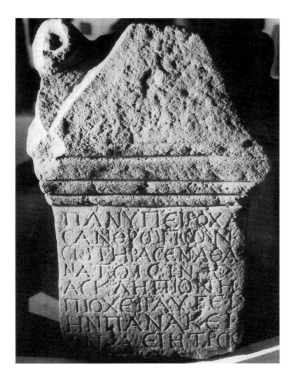

Figure 60 Altar from the second century AD, dedicated in Greek by the doctor Antiochus (62 cm×41 cm×18 cm). This was found near the presumed site of the hospital of the legionary fortress of the 20th legion at Deva (Chester, England). It is inscribed: 'The doctor Antiochus honours the all-surpassing saviour of men among the immortals, Asclepius of the gentle hands, Hygieia and Panacea...' (Photo supplied by Dr P Carrington and the Support Services Section, Grosvenor Museum, Chester, England)

At the Roman fort at Lanchester in County Durham, England, a bilingual doctor dedicated an altar to Aesculapius. The inscription on the front in Latin translates 'To Aesculapius Titanus Flavius, tribune, gladly and, willingly, and deservedly fulfilled his vow'; on the opposite side the dedication was repeated in Greek (Figure 61)[30].

A doctor named Marcus Aurelius... ocomas left a votive dedication slab depicting Aesculapius and his serpent-entwined staff with Salus at the Roman fort of Binchester in County Durham. This stated: 'To Aesculapius and Salus for the welfare of the Cavalry Regiment of Vettonians, Roman Citizens' (Figure 62)[31].

Another dedication to Aesculapius in Britain, inscribed only in Greek, was found at the Roman fort of Alauna at Maryport (Cumbria). This stated: 'To Asclepius Aulus Egnatius Pastor set this up' (RIB 808).

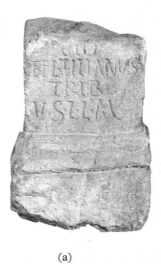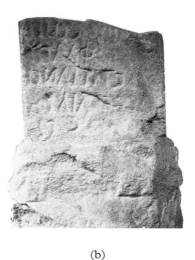

(a)   (b)

Figure 61 Altar from the Roman fort of Longovicium (30 cm×50 cm RIB 1072) (Lanchester, County Durham), dating to the late second century or third century AD. The inscription is bilingual
(a) The front bears a Latin inscription 'To Aesculapius Titanus Flavius, tribune, gladly and, willingly, and deservedly fulfilled his vow'
(b) The back has the same inscription written in Greek (Photos courtesy of Mr Richard Brickstock, Curator, Department of Archaeology and the Photographic Department, Archaeology Museum, University of Durham, England)

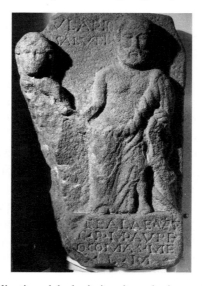

Figure 62 Votive dedication slab depicting Aesculapius and Salus from the Roman fort of Vinovia (40 cm×60 cm RIB 1028) (Binchester, County Durham, England), probably dating to the second century AD (Photo courtesy of Mr Richard Brickstock, Curator, Department of Archaeology and the Photographic Department, Archaeology Museum, University of Durham, England)

Birley found the most northern example of the spread of Greek influence by the Roman army. This was located at the legionary semi-fortress of Carpow on the banks of the River Tay in Perthshire, Scotland[32]. Here, part of a wine amphora with a graffito scratched in Greek has been found: 'ΠΡΑΣΓ' (Figure 63). Research showed that it had been added after firing.

Birley reported that Dioscorides gave a recipe for a wine flavoured with horehound which was deemed beneficial for the chest[33]. The damp Caledonian climate may well have contributed to coughs at this river side camp and the medical officer, a Greek doctor, had imported his own medicines from his native Greece.

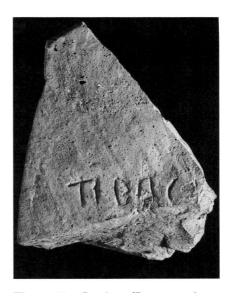

Figure 63 Greek graffito on amphora, labelling the contents horehound flavoured with wine; found at Carpow, Scotland and dated to 208–11 AD (© Trustees National Museums of Scotland)

The invasion of Scotland by Septimius Severus in 209 AD required the building of bridges over the Firth of Forth and the River Tay. Sir Charles Oman thought this feat was depicted on a coin of Severus showing a bridge of trestles supported by three galleys and approached by two ramps. Two emperors (Severus and Caracalla), four standard bearers and a horseman stand on the bridge and the waters below have waves like the sea[34]. It is possible that the bridge depicted on the coin was located at the site of the fort at Carpow[35].

Greek physicians of the Roman army gradually became romanized. This is demonstrated remarkably well by a dedication re-used in the jamb of a window in the nave of the church of Saint John the Baptist, Tunstall, Lancashire. The inscription uses Latin script but the author used the Greek spelling for Aesculapius and made a dedication to Hygieia rather than Salus (Figure 64). The re-used altar originated from the nearby Roman fort at Overborough.

Aesculapius and the native population of Britain
Aesculapius is likely to have been introduced to the native population of Britain as part of the gradual process of romanization, especially in towns and other places where romanization was taking place. In times

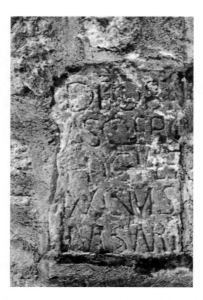

Figure 64   Part of an altar (20 cm×32.5 cm, RIB 609) inscribed in Roman script with Greek spelling of Aesculapius and the use of Hygieia in place of Salus. This inscription is in the west jamb of the easternmost window on the north wall of the Parish Church of Saint John the Baptist nave, Tunstall, Lancashire. The inscription reads: 'To the holy god Asclepius and to Hygieia, for the health of himself and of his own, Julius Saturninus' (Photo GDH with the kind permission of the Reverend Patrick Cotton)

of peace, the skills of the Greek *medici* were probably also available to the native people, and army physicians sometimes set up 'private practices' after discharge in the neighbourhood of their base camps. One of these might have been the donor of the Greek inscription at Chester reading: 'To the mighty Saviour Gods, I, Hermogenes, a doctor, set up this altar'. (RIB 461)

Two examples from the archaeological record suggest evidence for a native British awareness of Aesculapius. In chapter 2, reference was made to Hygieia acquiring an association with Athena who, in the Roman empire, became Salus acquiring an association with Minerva. This association is demonstrated at the sacred springs of two Celtic goddesses. At Coventina's Well (Carrawburgh, Northumbria), the native Celtic goddess was associated with a statue of Minerva and Aesculapius (Figure 14a). At Bath, the thermal springs of the native goddess Sulis became associated with Minerva at the elaborate Roman temple of Sulis Minerva. This is one of two temples known to have been built in classical style in the province of Britain.

At Corbridge, there is an altar associating the Celtic Goddess Brigantia with Jupiter and Salus. This is of interest because Brigantia

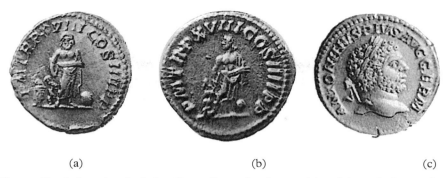

(a)   (b)   (c)

Figure 65 A denarius depicting Caracalla on the obverse (c) and Aesculapius on the reverse ((a) & (b)). This coin, dating to 213–7 AD, continues to be a relatively common type today and was the Aesculapius design copied by the London forger (Photo GDH)

was also a Celtic healing deity. The temple of Nodens at Lydney, Gloucestershire, was a unique late Romano-British temple built in the style of an Asclepian temple.

Romano-British coins are less subtle in their evidence for native knowledge and acceptance of Aesculapius. Clodius Albinus, a governor of Britain who, in 193 AD, accepted the title of 'Caesar' in exchange for supporting Septimius Severus during a period of civil war, minted coins depicting Aesculapius. Carausius, Commander of the Channel Fleet, declared himself Augustus in 286 AD and set up a local empire in Britain. He minted coins depicting Aesculapius at both of the known British mints; one of these is unique because it used a depiction of Aesculapius, rather than Salus, to accompany the inscription *Salus Aug* (Health to the Emperor).

An awareness of Aesculapius among the population of Roman Britain is inferred from the discovery of moulds used for producing forgeries of current coinage. These had been hurriedly discarded outside the site of 'Newgate' in the Roman Wall of London. The success of any such forgery depends on offering currency acceptable to commerce and non-gold coins require a design that will be accepted without attracting close scrutiny. In this case, the forger copied a coin of Caracalla in current circulation, which depicted Aesculapius on the reverse and Caracalla on the obverse (Figure 65)[36,37].

Summary
Archaeological findings, inscriptions, dedications, coins and medical instruments indicate that Greek doctors associated with the Roman army spread Aesculapius to the north-western limits of the Roman empire.

Notes and references

1. Some ancient authors who recorded the arrival of Asclepius in Rome include: Valerius Maximus in *Facta and Dicta Memorabilia* I, 8, 2 (ET 848), who described the event in detail and added the serpent swimming to the island; Livy in *Periocha* XI (ET 846); Anonymus in *de Viris Illustribus* 22, 1–3 (ET 849); Claudius in *de Consulatu Stilichonis* III, 171–3 (ET 851); and Arnobius in *Adversus Nationales* VII, 44–8 (ET 852).

2. This reflects the change of Asclepius' status in the ancient world. Apollo, himself, controlled the epidemic of Rome in 432 BC. His replacement by Asclepius in Greece was recorded in earlier chapters; the reference to the oracle of Delphi referring the city fathers of Rome to Epidaurus was the ultimate stamp of approval for Asclepius.

3. Ovid's account exaggerated the traditional need of a serpent from Epidaurus to establish a new sanctuary. He used poetic licence to enhance the stature of Rome when describing Asclepius' change of residence from Epidaurus to Rome.

4. There has been some debate as to whether or not Antium already had a temple to Asclepius or if the temple of Apollo was converted after this visit.

5. This was a description of the elaborate 'religio' ceremony needed for the addition of a powerful, new foreign deity to the Roman pantheon.

6. The figure on the front deck of the ship has been interpreted as a helmsman steering the ship, however, this would not be possible with the type of vessel depicted. The figure was more likely to be the ancient equivalent of today's river pilot who directs the master of the vessel into the safe channels.

7. de Roquefeuil, S. *Le serpent d'Asclepios-Esculape, Paris*. Extrait du catalogue de l'exposition. Le Bestaire, Hôtel de la Monnie, Juin–Septembre 1974.

8. Watts D. *Christians and pagans in Roman Britain*. London: Routledge, 1991.

9. Woodward A. *Shrines and sacrifice*. London: English Heritage, 1992.

10. The marshes of Rome were home to the malaria-transmitting *Anopheles* mosquito.

11. The Tiber, like the rivers flowing through great cities of today, was liable to flooding. Several floods have been recorded on the island; the last one submerged the main courtyard of the hospital by three feet and the nave of the church of San Bartolomeo by eight feet. This probably reflects the architectural accuracy of the ancient vessel; the 'deck' of the bow was five feet below the 'deck' of the stern. The direction of the ship is interesting: if the bow, with its pointed shape, faced the current as the tide-breaks of bridge abutments do, then there would have been less erosion at the bow and water would have been deflected away from the sides of the island. A rounded stern facing the current of the Tiber would have done the opposite. Kerenyi suggested that the east-west axis was associated with Apollo and the sun. The church of San Bartolomeo has its sanctuary and altar at the west end of the church. This is in contrast to traditional church orientation in Britain and other countries where the altar was located at the eastern end of the church that not only allowed the worshippers to face Jerusalem but also allowed in light for morning services[13].

12. Kerenyi C. *Asklepios*. Bollinger Series LXV 3. Pantheon Books, 1959.

13. Whitman WB. Rome's Tiber island. *MD* December 1992: 25–9.

14. Forbes SR. The Regia. *Archaeological J* 1901; **LVIII**: 142–3.

15. Lewis P, ed. *An illustrated history of medicine*. Middlesex: Hamlyn Publishing Group, 1968: 76.

16. Penn RG. *Medicine on ancient Greek and Roman coins*. London: L Seaby and BT Batsford, 1994.

17. Alternative healthcare systems that maintain their own professional standards, such as chiropractic and homoeopathic medicine, are available today.

18. Nutton V. *Archiatri and the medical profession in antiquity*. Papers at the British School at Rome 1977; **45**: 191–226.

19. Jackson R. *Doctors and diseases in the Roman empire*. London: British Museum Press, 1988: 57.

20. Webster G. *The Roman imperial army*. London: Adam and Charles Black, 1969.

21. Richmond IA. The Roman army medical service. *Medical Gazette* (Durham University) 1952; **46**(3): 2–6.

22. Under the Roman republic, legionary soldiers retired with a gratuity in the form of a land grant. In 13 BC, Augustus replaced the land grant with a monetary payment for soldiers who had normally served 20 years.

23. (a) Pitts LF, St Joseph JK. *Inchtuthill*. London: Britannia Monographs, 1985.
    (b) Richmond IA. The hospital, Inchtuthill. *J Roman Studies* 1986; **XLV**: 91–3.

24. Photographs of the site, taken by Dr Colin Martin of the University of St Andrews, Scotland, further elaborate the details of Professor Richmond's[23] provisional interpretation of the site. [Personal communication.]

25. Gilson A. A doctor at Housesteads. *Archaeologia Aeliana* 1976; **5**: 164–5.

26. Jackson R. *Doctors and diseases in the Roman empire*. London: British Museum Press, 1988: 82.

27. (a) Nutton V. Medicine and the Roman army; a further reconsideration. *Med Hist* 1969; **13**: 260–70.
    (b) Scarborough J. Roman medicine and the legions: a reconsideration. *Med Hist* 1969; **13**: 254–61.

28. Forrest M, Hughes M. *The Romans discover Britain*. Cambridge School Classics Project, Classical Studies 13-6. Cambridge: Press Syndicate of the University of Cambridge, 1988: 47.

29. Nutton V. A Greek doctor at Chester. *J Chester Archaeol Soc* 1968; **55**: 7–13.

30. RIB Longovicium, Lanchester (County Durham): 1072.

31. RIB Vinovia, Binchester (County Durham): 1028.

32. Wright RP. Roman Britain 1962. *J Roman Studies* 1963; **53**: 166.

33. Birley RE. Excavations of the Roman fort at Carpow, Perthshire, 1961–1962. *PSAS* 1963–4; **96**: 202.

34. The bridge was probably supported by more than three boats but the artist was constrained by the coin size. A similar bridge appears on a coin minted by Marcus Aurelius to commemorate his crossing of the Danube. Sir Charles Oman stated that the toil of bridge building necessary for the invasion of Scotland exhausted the army (*Numismatic Chronicle*, 5th series 1931; **11**: 137).

35. Further interpretation of the significance of bridges on Severan coins has been reviewed by AS Robertson in: Robertson AS. Roman frontier studies. In: Hanson WS, Keppie LFJ, eds. *BAR International* series 71(1), Oxford, 1979. In her review, Robertson identifies the medallion that is in the Cabinet des Médailles, Paris; she describes it as an occasional or special issue bronze 'as' or a small medallion minted by Caracalla in 209 AD. Robertson feels it represents the crossing of any great river during the Severan Campaign and favours the Tay at Carpow as the model used by the artist. A point in favour of the Firth of Forth as the site is the size of the waves depicted on the water. It is possible that the stress and hardships of the campaign even exceeded the powers of Aesculapius and Apollo Granno, contributing to the death of Severus at York in 211 AD.

36. The spread of Aesculapius by the Roman army is demonstrated by a coin dated 213–7 AD portraying Caracalla on the obverse and Aesculapius on the reverse

(Figure 65). An exhibit at the Museum of London, London Wall, London, shows a similar coin and tells the following story: 'One of these genuine coins together with the molds for forgeries of similar coins were found in a garbage dump at the base of the turret at Newgate on the Roman Wall of London. One of these depicted Caracalla on the obverse and Aesculapius on the reverse. The coins were thought to have been discarded hurriedly by a forger who was being pursued by the authorities; their find resulted in dating the enlargement of the Roman Wall of the City of London to between 190 and 200 AD.

37. Emperor Severus and his two sons, Geta and Caracalla, brought their armies to Britain in 209 AD to re-establish Roman authority and civic order. These emperors favoured Aesculapius and depicted him on the reverse of many of their coins. His depiction also symbolized health for the emperor and the Roman state. During this time, Aesculapius was the favourite god and his popularity with emperors must have both boosted his popularity with the army and introduced him further to the civilian population of Roman Britain.

Chapter 8

Medical practice by Greek and Roman physicians

Greek physicians influenced medical practice throughout antiquity. Until the fifth century BC, sickness was considered a manifestation of divine displeasure and Asclepian temple medicine evolved from the propitiation of Asclepius. During this century, Hippocrates and his followers developed the concept that disease resulted from physical causes and their clinical observations led to empirical knowledge about sickness and health. In 292 BC, Asclepius was adopted as Aesculapius, the Roman god of medicine, and Greek medical practices spread to Rome. Doctors brought Aesculapius to parts of the Roman empire that did not already have a Greek heritage (see chapter 7). The prosperity and politics of the Roman world facilitated further growth of medical skills and techniques.

Asclepius was the common thread weaving continuity between these epochs of classical medicine. Physicians believed Asclepius guided their work and that their patron god had discovered the skills of medical practice, preparation of drugs and surgery (ET 355 & 356).

> 'For I have achieved perfection in the medical art, in spite of the fact that I have already reached old age. Indeed, not even the discoverer of this art, Asclepius, did so. . . .' Hippocrates, *Epistulae*, 20 (ET 349)

Asclepiad medical care
Asclepiads recognized that their abilities had limitations and, although they were not directly involved with temple medicine, considered the incubation ritual to be a 'friendly ally rather than the hated enemy of their craft'[1].

Before the fifth century BC, temple medicine was a purely religious ritual. It is reasonable to speculate that temple priests gradually realized that physicians' skills could be a valuable adjunct to their own, especially when treating supplicants unable or unwilling to stay for the incubation ritual. The fame of Hippocrates and the Hippocratic school attracted patients to Cos, which probably facilitated the priests' departure from their early rigid orthodoxy. Prayers and ritual of the Asclepieion were combined with medical therapy.

Collaboration between priest and physician

It is not possible to give a precise date for the hypothetical, informal alliance of the theurgical practices of priests with the medical skills of the Asclepiads. Support for this collaboration is demonstrated by the coin of Epidaurus, minted in 323–240 BC, depicting an altar on which a *thymiaterion* (incense burner) was flanked by two cupping vessels (Figure 31). This coin is testimony to the alliance, repudiating historians who have argued that physicians were completely segregated from Asclepian temple therapy[2,3]. Ancient sculptors recorded this alliance between priest and practitioner. A sculpted stone in the Athenian Asclepieion depicts cupping vessels flanking a case of surgical instruments (Figure 38). In the Athens National Museum, a bas-relief depicts Asclepius or a doctor treating a patient's shoulder by cupping and incision, while the background shows a duplicate portrait of the patient asleep in the *abaton*, with his shoulder being licked by a serpent. The standard interpretation of this bas-relief is that a temple serpent treated the patient while he dreamt that Asclepius was responsible. An alternative view is that medical treatment had been started by a physician but was completed by Asclepius' serpent during the incubation ritual (Figure 66). An extant fragment of another bas-relief from Athens portrays a doctor operating on a patient's head with Asclepius, depicted in the background, supervising the procedure — this is similar to today's consultant supervising surgery performed by a junior doctor.

The tablets recording winners of the medical competitions during the festival of Asclepius at Ephesus were described in chapter 4. These also indicate that the Asclepieia supported and encouraged medical research. Physicians were attracted to the Asclepieia by the many pilgrims willing to supplement their divine care with temporal therapy. Physicians accepted the recommendations for incubation with the same alacrity they accepted fees for their own contribution to treatment. Many supplicants came to the temples to pray for their own continued good health or for the health of loved ones. Some sought primary care from temple priests; others came because they suffered complex and complicated problems that their local physicians could not treat. The Asclepiads probably referred difficult problems to the temple so patients could benefit from conservative (expectant) therapy, nootherapy, reassurance and healing by touch. In addition, the 'second opinion' of Asclepius would verify the complexity of the case and confirm the

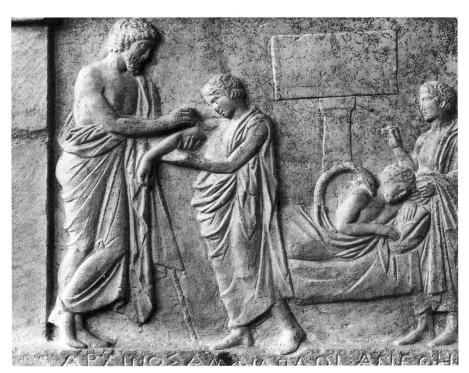

Figure 66   Bas-relief (c400–350 BC) of a patient receiving treatment to his shoulder at the temple. The god has been described as Asclepius but the inscription records that the patient, Archinos, has given the dedication to Amphiaraus, an identical healing deity located at Oropos who gained favour during the Peloponnesian Wars. The double depiction of the patient indicates on the left the patient dreaming of a physician or the god holding a cupping vessel in his left hand and about to incise and drain the anterior axilla while on the right the same patient is undergoing the abaton ritual with the temple serpent healing the shoulder (Photo © National Archaeological Museum, Athens, Greece)

doctor's competence and reputation. Despite this tacit collaboration, Asclepiad medical care remained independent from temple medicine. Today, we have patients who combine 'alternate medicine' with standard medical therapy.

The clustering of physicians at Asclepian centres was useful when discussing patients under their care. Their interchange of ideas and experiences contributed to the on-going learning experience of clinical medicine and was the ancient counterpart of 'medical rounds', 'continuing medical education' and 'maintenance of competence'.

Hippocratic school and clinical medicine
Hippocrates was the first physician to record detailed history of a patient's illness and his accurate records became the building blocks of

clinical diagnosis. This system of detection continues to be used by physicians today, who assess a new patient or a different illness by extensive inquiry into the details and sequence of symptoms as well as details about past health, occupation, family diseases and lifestyle. The resulting complete patient history contains clues leading the doctor to a differential and provisional diagnosis (see chapter 12).

Jones and Potter, the modern translators of *The Hippocratic corpus*, have concluded that most of its contents were not actually written by Hippocrates (as discussed in chapter 2)[4,5]. However, his fame was such that he became a clinical and literary legend; readers of today should mentally place 'Hippocratic school' in parentheses behind the writings credited to him.

The Hippocratic school divided a disease course into three stages. First, an imbalance of body humours (liquids) caused by internal or external factors. Second, the reaction of the body to the altered balance by producing a fusion (coction) such that none of the humours are left in excess and the pain and symptoms are relieved. This process was accompanied by heat production (fever) similar to that generated during normal digestion, and involved digestion and absorption of food, production of the humours and their excretion if in excess — it produced a feeling of warmth. Fever due to infection was a common problem; without the benefit of a clinical thermometer, clinical details of fever patterns recorded in the Hippocratic writings are diagnostic of malaria! Hippocratic physicians recorded and studied the patterns of warmth in much the same way as today's study of temperature charts, and their interpretation often gave a correct prognosis for the course of the patient's illness whether it be recovery or death. The final phase was a resultant 'crisis' with discharge of the residual excessive humour (via blood, phlegm, vomit, faeces, urine or sweat). A successful crisis was followed by improvement while an ineffective crisis resulted in death[4-6]. If nature was unable to use the ordinary methods of evacuation, then excessive humour accumulated in one part of the body and produced a localized swelling or tumour; this demonstrated signs of inflammation, redness and warmth. Such localization is clinically known today as a boil or abscess which will subsequently point and discharge pus, or which needs artificial drainage by an incision. The Hippocratic aphorism '*ubi pus evacuo*' (I drain pus wherever it is) remains a basic tenet of medical practice.

This tripartite theory of disease created a world of medical thought with unlimited horizons. When the cause of sickness was released from the shackles of superstition relating to displeasure of the gods, physicians began their long voyage of medical discoveries. Their theory on the pathogenesis of disease summarizes our present knowledge of the onset of infection; this is influenced by external or internal sources of organisms whose virulence may be modified by the patient's internal resistance and by immunity which is manifest by the patient's immune and inflammatory response. Internal resistance is lowered by a variety of factors including fatigue, malnutrition, exposure, stress and the presence of other debilitating illness. Immunity may be passively improved by generations of racial exposure or by an individual's previous exposure to infections. Today, active immunization by vaccines has eradicated previously fatal diseases such as smallpox, polio and measles[6].

Before the antibiotic era, streptococcal (pneumococcal) pneumonia and other infections followed a course of crisis frequently preceded by a discharge of liquefied residual of infection such as sputum and profuse sweats. Failure to have a satisfactory crisis resulted in death.

When the Asclepiads practised medicine according to the teachings of Hippocrates and his followers, they sought a physical cause for the imbalance of the body humours which resulted in illness. In using methods to correct this imbalance, they would have followed the dictums contained in section 7 of Hippocrates' final aphorism:

'Those [diseases] which drugs do not cure are cured by surgery; those which surgery does not cure are cured by cauterisation; those which cauterisation does not cure must be considered incurable.'[7]

Balancing the body humours
The doctrine of the four humours was based on the ideas of the Greek philosopher Empedocles of Acragas, Sicily (c490–430 BC), who believed that all matter was formed from four ultimate, unchangeable elements — fire, water, air and earth — which possessed the characteristics of hot, cold, dry and moist[8]. Using this concept of matter, Hippocrates formulated the theory that the body was constituted from four humours, each containing two of Empedocles' basic characteristics: these were black bile (cold and dry characteristics); yellow bile (warm and dry); blood (warm and moist) and phlegm (cold and moist). A state of health existed when the humours were in balance, while illness resulted from excess or deficiency of one or more of the humours.

Hippocrates' concept of yellow bile as an elemental body fluid merits further clinical elaboration. Bile is a yellow digestive fluid containing pigments that originate from breakdown products of haemoglobin. It is formed in the liver and excreted into the duodenum;

it is also concentrated in the gall bladder where it becomes more viscous and darker in colour (black bile). As a result of cupping (discussed in detail below), Hippocratic physicians had an opportunity to observe the clotting of blood and would have noticed that the process is accompanied by the appearance of a yellow fluid (serum). It would have been difficult for them not to conclude that the fluid component of blood was anything but yellow bile. It is probable that Hippocratic yellow bile included both plasma (non-cellular component of blood) and serum (yellow fluid seen after blood has clotted).

Hippocratic physicians advocated treatments that corrected, by various means, the imbalance of the four humours. Regulation of diet was very important as some foods by nature were warmer than others and produced more bile, while cooler foods produced more phlegm. Excess yellow bile was removed by emetics, cupping, harsh laxatives and possibly by enemas. Dry cupping and expectorants removed excess phlegm. Excess blood was removed by wet cupping. Different drinks and waters from various springs were used to correct excess of 'dry'. Clystering (enemas) was used to expurgate waste, excess moist and dry. Persistent constipation is a common complaint of elderly, debilitated or immobilized patients due to a bulky, dry, hard stool producing various pains and symptoms. It is treated by enemas; refractory cases require a three 'H' enema meaning 'high, hot and a hell of a lot'!

The ancients' corrections of imbalances between moist and dry humours have modern counterparts. Restoring fluid balance by intravenous or oral means remains the basic treatment for diarrhoea, vomiting and fever regardless of the cause. Similarly with respiratory problems, phlegm may be too watery (moist) as in pulmonary oedema. Treatment may involve removing blood or administering medicines to increase fluid excretion by the kidneys. Some respiratory conditions result from a deficiency of 'moist' causing thick, tenacious sputum of asthma or the dry, non-productive cough of croup and other chest ailments; excess 'dry' in the lungs may be corrected by moist inhalations and expectorant mixtures.

Cystitis (inflammation of the bladder) is the most common urinary problem with symptoms of the frequent urge to urinate and the passing of small amounts of urine accompanied by burning. These symptoms suggest an imbalance of moist and warm humours, needing an increased intake of cold fluids and the ingestion of foods producing coolness. Before antibiotics were synthesized, cystitis was treated with high fluid intake and medicines to alkalize or acidify urine. One of today's most popular folk remedies for the bladder is consumption of large volumes of cranberry juice.

Hippocratic physicians observed urine output and noted its clarity, odour and taste. Even today, urine testing is an important part of many treatments and its colour, clarity and odour are still noted. Testing for sugar, albumen and cells is an integral component of medical assessment; fortunately, tasting has been replaced by a simple 'dipstick' test. Fluids continue to be pushed and foods regulated in accordance with the results of urinalysis.

It is interesting to speculate whether or not Hippocratic physicians recognized the differences between vomitus containing black or yellow bile, and the mixtures of the two. It is probable that they misinterpreted melaena or black stools (due to an upper gastro-intestinal haemorrhage) as being due to an excess of black bile alone and may have inappropriately prescribed cupping. Jaundice would be an easily recognized condition due to excess bile; today, its degree is measured by a direct and indirect bilirubin test which differentiates between obstructive and non-obstructive jaundice, ie jaundice due to black or yellow bile or a mixture of the two. The patient's skin would have provided a variety of signs allowing inclusion into the underlying humoral theory. Skin may be hot and dry with fevers, but also moist with sweating as evidence of the crisis. It may be flushed and hot suggesting excess blood, or dry and scaly indicating an underlying deficiency of moist humours. It may also be yellow with jaundice (an excess of yellow bile), pale or sallow with a deficiency of blood and show excess redness (rubor) with too much blood.

The Hippocratic concept of disease contained principles that apply to present-day haematology. Anaemic blood demonstrates an excess ratio of plasma or serum to red blood cells, representing to Hippocratic physicians an imbalance of 'dry' and 'moist' properties of the warm humours ie yellow bile and blood. Blood from a patient with dehydration or polycythaemia demonstrates a visible and measurable excess of red blood cells to plasma, ie an imbalance of blood to yellow bile. Treatment of these conditions follows the broad principles of the humoral theory. Severe acute anaemia may be treated by a transfusion of packed red blood cells while dehydration (an excess of dry over moist) is treated by oral or intravenous fluids. Polycythaemia (an excess of warm moist humour over cold moist humour) is treated by venesection (removal of blood by incision into a vein).

Hippocratic physicians believed blood was formed in the liver. This theory is only correct for foetal blood formation although the body may revert to hepatic blood formation at times of severe haematological stress. Liver and splenic enlargement described in some Hippocratic case histories were probably manifestations of thalassaemia; this is a congenital anaemia occurring in the Mediterranean region and is accompanied by blood formation in the liver (extramedullary haematopoiesis). These physicians treated an excess of blood by wet cupping which required a venesection using a cupping vessel for removal or a simple bowl for collecting.

Hippocrates expanded
The humoral theory influenced medical treatment for many centuries. Although multiple medical advances superseded its use, it was brilliant in its conception. Modern medicine has rediscovered that the body is influenced by a variety of opposing forces and that a state of health is often dependent on this balance. The number of medical conditions caused by an imbalance of new 'humoral factors' is increasing at an exponential rate. A few examples are noted below.

- An excess of low-density lipoprotein cholesterol to high-density lipoprotein cholesterol causes atherosclerosis and heart disease. Diet and medications correct the imbalance and arrest progress of the condition, as well as improving circulation and symptoms.
- An imbalance and activation of starter and inhibitor genes favour the development of cancer. Cancer research is attempting to find methods to counteract the process.
- An imbalance of lymphocyte types results in inability to combat infection and facilitates the development of certain tumours. Therapy aims to restore the correct lymphocyte balance.

Regulation of hormone levels, blood clotting and many other body diseases requires internal balance. Newer treatment strategies are being developed, in particular for blocking the action or uptake of disease-producing factors.

Cupping
Greek and Roman physicians used wet cupping to remove excess warm and moist humour (blood). The modern term for this procedure is a venesection. Cupping vessels became the physician's hallmark from the fourth century BC to the 19th century AD and were depicted on coins, bas-reliefs and art (Figures 31 & 38). The cupping instrument (*curcubitula*) was a bell-shaped appliance made of glass, horn or bronze; this was heated and applied over an incision that had been made into a vein. When the hot air inside the vessel cooled, a vacuum was created that sucked out blood, the volume of which could be

measured and controlled. This suction method could also be applied to the drainage of an abscess or boil.

An alternative method of bloodletting was to make an incision over a large superficial vein and to collect the blood into a special bleeding bowl. The Louvre Museum in Paris displays a fifth century BC Attic vase depicting the procedure, which continued until the late 19th century when blood was collected in specially shaped bowls. These 'barber surgeon's bowls' had a concave notch in the rim so they could be applied to the side of the neck under a large superficial vein incision. In the 20th century, this technique was replaced by the insertion into a vein of a large bore hollow needle connected to a syringe. In the 1960s, however, modern medicine rediscovered the Greek physicians' simplicity of the vacuum principle for removing small or large volumes of blood. Small amounts of blood are needed for a variety of diagnostic tests, and are now collected in different types of vacuum tubes through a small bore needle with an adapter — this allows the simple collection of multiple samples. The vacuum tubes have eliminated the previous painful experience of blood testing. A large bore needle or trochar, connected via a flexible tube to a vacuum bottle, is used for collecting larger volumes of blood from donors or patients undergoing a therapeutic venesection for polycythaemia[9,10].

The cupping vessel was also used to produce a localized area of counter irritation (dry cupping). This procedure required no incision. The vessel was positioned over the area to be treated where an increased supply of blood was sucked; this produced local warmth and redness as well as more white blood cells, resulting in pain relief and hastened healing. Even today, physicians occasionally see patients from the Mediterranean with a circular bruise mark at the site of their symptoms, indicating a trial of home-therapy with cupping before visiting the doctor.

Galen

Galen (129–210 AD) was the best known physician from the Roman era. He was a teacher, writer, pharmacist, physiologist, anatomist surgeon and physician. His contributions to medicine were immense and, for centuries, he remained the ultimate authority in western and Islamic medicine. The significance of his belief in Asclepius is briefly summarized.

Galen was born at Pergamum of Greek ancestry. He qualified in both medicine and philosophy after studying at Pergamum and Alexandria for 12 years. His early practice with the treatment of gladiators provided him with expert knowledge of anatomy and developed his surgical skills. He settled in Rome in 162 AD and, although he became the most renowned Greek *medicus* in Rome, remained a follower of Asclepius: '... the ancestral god Asclepius, whose servant I declared myself to be; for he saved me when I was suffering from a deadly condition of an abscess.' *De Libris Propriis*, II (ET 458)

He referred to the Asclepiads in his book *De Anatomicis Administrationibus* (ET 229): 'So the art of medicine passed beyond the family of Asclepiads and it subsequently grew worse as it passed through successive generations; people needed to have something written down, so they could rely on accurate theoretical knowledge. For in the old days, it was not considered necessary to undertake anatomical studies, or even have books dealing with such matters.'

In this statement, Galen seems to be rationalizing his medical writings while confirming his loyalty to his belief in Asclepius. He is acknowledging the need for knowledge of anatomy and the evolution of medical methods beyond those developed by Hippocrates. Galen believed that talking to patients and obtaining their histories was important. He incorporated the four humours into a system of personality assessment; the descriptive terms he used have survived in today's vocabulary with the terms 'melancholic', 'choleric', 'phlegmatic' and 'sanguine'.

He had a shrewd attitude towards cupping and advocated the removal of only a small amount of blood. He probably had doubts about internal bleeding being due to an excess of blood and his attitude is a contrast to the excesses of the 16th to 19th centuries during which bleeding often aggravated the symptoms and hastened patient death. Galen described the treatment of fractures, dislocations and resection of bone; his technique for emergency limb amputation was still practised by army surgeons during World War One. He studied pharmacology and was the first to experiment with physiology, associating the kidneys with urine formation, and to assign a role to the spleen which was mainly to remove black bile from the blood. He studied the effects of various parts of the gastrointestinal tract on ingested food and the effect of digested food on the four humours. He recognized innate body heat suggesting knowledge of the heat- and energy-producing processes of metabolism. He was the first to propose a connection between arteries and veins, but developed only a very limited concept of circulation[11]. He wrote several treatises and many of those surviving were still accepted into the 18th century as the ultimate authority on medicine, pharmacology, physiology and surgery.

Pharmacology

Graeco-Roman physicians used a variety of medications from plant, mineral and animal sources. One of the earliest drugs available was *terra sigillata* (sealed earth) which initially came from the Mediterranean island of Lemnos in c500 BC. It was excavated here from a hillside once a year in the presence of civic and religious dignitaries[12]. The clay was washed and refined, then formed into pastilles and sun-dried[12]. These trochets contained silica, kaolin, aluminium, chalk and magnesia which have good adsorbent properties and are useful in relieving diarrhoeal symptoms and indigestion; the modern North American proprietary products Amphojel, Maalox and Rolaids have similar properties. Galen visited Lemnos on two occasions and it is likely that he knew about *terra sigillata* and its special adsorptive properties. Perhaps he wished to experiment with a constipating agent possessing specific adsorptive properties for body humours. A recent addition to the physician's armamentarium is cholestyramine resin, a medication used to remove bile acid (yellow bile) from the intestinal tract with a constipating effect.

Hippocratic physicians prescribed from a pharmacopoeia of more than 300 remedies. These included: hellebore which was used for its carminative and emetic actions to balance the body humours, silphium (asafoetida), wine, parsley and many other drugs which continued to be prescribed until the beginning of the 20th century (Figure 67). Wine was used as a medicine; the Aminean variety from northern Italy was recommended for diarrhoea and the common cold. An amphora inscribed 'AMINE' was found near the hospital site of the legionary fortress of Caerleon, South Wales[13]. Wine was also recommended in the Roman fort at South Shields, Durham, England, where a grey wine jar was found with the inscription in Greek: 'Be healthy, drink'. One wonders whether or not Publius Viboleius Secundus,

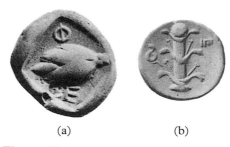

(a)   (b)

Figure 67
(a) A bud of hellebore (or a grain of wheat in a husk) on the reverse of a coin of Pherae (c400 BC) (Photo BMC, M&W)
(b) A coin from Cyrenaica depicting the silphium plant and a serpent. This was the symbol used on the reverse of coins from Cyrenaica from the sixth century BC until 60 BC, when uncontrolled harvesting resulted in its extinction. Dioscorides described an Asian variety of silphium, in addition to the one from Cyrenaica. The variety from Cyrenaica was preferred for medical therapy (Photo BMC, M&W)

who erected a votive altar to Aesculapius at the east gate of the fort, had also imported the wine[14a]. Greek and Roman physicians discovered the value of wine as an antiseptic[14b] and as a vehicle for medications (modern pharmacists continue to formulate prescriptions of elixirs containing up to 20% alcohol). In addition to the topical and oral routes, medications were sometimes inhaled as snuff.

Silphium, 'food of the gods' or 'devil's dung', was an interesting drug derived from an unusual plant native to Cyrenaica. The plant became the symbol of Cyrenaica and was depicted on the reverse of its coins; a small serpent sometimes accompanied the depiction, indicating its medicinal use. Uncontrolled exploitation resulted in extinction of this species (Figure 67b). The active ingredients are salicylic acid and volatile oils; it was prescribed for the treatment of asthma, bronchitis or sore throat and used as a carminative in flatulent colic, as a laxative and as a stimulant to the brain.

Scribonius Largus, a physician who 'lived a soldier-like life' by travelling, collected plant and herbal data from around the world. He wrote the first modern pharmacopoeia, *Compositiones*[13,15], (43–8 AD) and agreed with Herophilus, the Alexandrian physician, who said drugs are like 'divine hands' because they produce effects like a divine touch. Largus was the first to recognize that different patients have varying constitutions and not all compounds suit everyone. Therefore, the dosage of drugs had to be individualized. He could also be called 'the father of clinical pharmacology' as he felt that only physicians with clinical experience should prescribe drugs. Dioscorides was a physician who travelled with the Roman armies. He collected data on 600 plants, 30 animal products and 90 minerals. The information obtained was used to improve the health of the Roman army and it is possible that he discovered the value of dock leaves for the treatment of scurvy[16]. His book *De Materia Medica* (50–70 AD), which describes medicines and the rules for their collection, storage and preparation, remained for 1,600 years as the ultimate authority on the subject. Although copies of it were rare, legionary physicians as well as other physicians who had visited the major medical libraries at Pergamum, Cos, Ephesus, Epidaurus, Rome, Athens and Alexandria must have divulged parts of its contents to their confrères. This is supported by the finding of one of Dioscorides' preparations at the legionary fortress on the banks of the Firth of Tay at Carpow in Scotland.

Galen the pharmacist
Galen's work with the compounding of drugs has earned him the title 'the father of polypharmacy'. For centuries, 'galenicals' were the

cornerstone of pharmacological practice. Standard medical preparations (as an extract or tincture), containing one or more active constituents of a plant made by a process leaving the inert and other undesirable constituents of the plant undissolved, are today called galenicals. He wrote 30 books related to pharmacy and his prescriptions for the use of hellebore, hyoscyamus and colocynth remained state of the art until the 18th century. His most enduring prescription was one for a cold cream, the formula of which is still used by physicians and is contained in most modern cosmetic cold creams[12]. He conceived broad principles for drug action and tried to relate them to their affinity for body humours with subsequent stimulatory or neutralizing actions. He also related drug actions to their effects on hot/cold and dry/moist qualities within the body with a secondary effect on contraction and relaxation. He had a special interest in cathartics (laxatives) with specificity for drawing out excess or defective humours.

Galen believed in individualized dosage designed to give maximum therapeutic effect with minimum side-effects. This represented a major advance on the prescription for snake bite recorded in verse on a stone in the temple of Asclepius at Cos:

'Take 2 denarii of wild thyme, and the same quantity of opopanax and bearwort (*meum*) respectively; 1 denarius of trefoil seed; and of aniseed, fennel seed, ammi and parsley, 6 denarii respectively, with 12 denarii of meal of fitches.' the Elder Pliny, *Natural History*, XX, 24 (100), 264 (ET 796)

The denarius was a Roman silver coin with a weight varying with economic conditions. This prescription reveals that the Elder Pliny was not a numismatist and the results of this prescription may have varied with the date of the coin used[17]!

Pharmacist's equipment
Greek and Roman physicians used balance scales, pestle and mortar, flasks and pharmacy bowls that sometimes had the name 'Asclepius' inscribed around the rim. They also used the spatula probe (*spathomele*) which had a rounded finial at the narrow end and a flat spatula at the opposite end. This probe could be used clinically to explore cavities or sinuses and was employed pharmacologically to mix medications. The spatula end was multi-functional, used to spread or remove medications and served as a curette, cautery, blunt dissector and even a tongue depressor. Until recently, pharmacists used an ordinary wooden tongue depressor to transfer and fill their jars with

ointments and creams! The *spathomele* had the potential for multiple exposures to contamination and probably contributed to the spread of many infections. *Lingulae* were long, thin instruments designed to remove medications or cosmetics from small-necked containers, but used as tongue depressors.

Unadulterated medications were stored in sealed containers, many of which were works of art with elaborately decorated labels. The most frequently used drugs were carried in small, bronze boxes with internal compartments and a secure sliding lid. Drugs were compounded on ground-stone slabs, such as one with a worn surface discovered in Colchester and now displayed in its museum.

Liquid medicines were sometimes dispensed from a glass jug with a spout shaped like a dropper, and morphine was placed in special vials shaped like a poppy leaf. These designs warned an illiterate user of the potency of the product, similar to the notched blue-glass coffin bottles of the early 20th century. A second or third century AD prescription from Kenchester, England, for an ointment of 'poppy' (morphine), recommended after an attack of inflammation of the eyes, was a prototype of today's topical anaesthetic ointment. Roman physicians sometimes carried dispensing tools on a chatelaine such as the one found at Corbridge holding a *lingula*, forceps, probe and scoop[18]. The pharmacological armamentarium of the Greek and Roman physicians remained state of the art for the next 15 centuries while dispensing pharmacists of the first one-half of the 20th century still used similar equipment and many of the same preparations.

Surgical instruments and procedures

Greek and Roman physicians developed a versatile range of surgical instruments, some of which were probably adapted from tools already in use by carpenters, masons and metal workers. As they were made from bronze, many, except for any iron or wooden components, have been preserved in a variety of geological environments ranging from the desert sands, volcanic ashes of Pompeii to the clay and chalky soils of Britain (Figure 68). It was common practice to make instruments serving a double function; even today, the handle of a scalpel may be used as a blunt instrument to separate layers of tissue. The 'Coudee-type' forceps from Longborough, England, had a serpent-headed handle allowing it to function as a probe. Many instruments had customized handles, grooved or ridged to assist intricate manipulation in the operative field; those serving a dual function were made so they could be held in the middle[18]. The ready availability of skilled metal workers facilitated modification and improvement in design, resulting

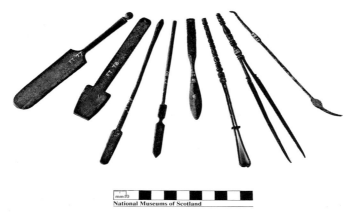

Figure 68   Medical instruments from Cramond, Scotland, dating to the second or third century AD. Cautery instruments with (from left to right): i) spatula-shaped end with a width of 2 cm ii) sawn-off spatula-shaped end with a width of 1.45cm iii) the end has chamfered edges with width of 9–6mm and the handle has an olivary tip which helped balance the instrument and could be used for cautery iv) the end is chamfered and terminates in a point. Scalpel handle shaped for firm grasp v) a slot for detachable scalpel blades vi) tissue forceps with interlocking teeth and a ring-lock vii) dissecting forceps terminating in a blunt round point viii) lingula used for withdrawing medications either for local application or for preparing prescriptions (Photograph courtesy of the Trustees of the National Museums of Scotland ©)

in a remarkably modern-looking series of surgical instruments developed by the first century AD. Such instruments allowed major advances in operative treatment.

Probes were used to separate tendons, arteries, veins and nerves and to drain pus from the sinuses of deep abscesses (facilitating the Hippocratic adage '*ubi pus evacuo*'). They also had double-ended probes (*specilla*) of various shapes and sizes, enabling them to explore wounds, body passages and fistulae and, by the sense of feel, to determine the state of underlying tissues. This information, combined with their clinical experience, enabled them to form a mental image of the underlying pathology and plan appropriate therapy. Today's surgeon has, of course, the benefit of 'hard copy' information based on X-rays, ultrasounds and tomograms.

Exploration for bladder stones used slightly longer instruments, some of which were especially shaped to facilitate intrauterine examination. Hippocratic physicians advocated the use of these instruments for the evacuation of pus from the uterus. Soranus described their value in plugging the external cervical os of the uterus at a time of severe haemorrhage. The late Dr Calvin Wells described a Roman uterine sound found in Norfolk which could have been used to rupture the amniotic membrane around a foetus to produce abortion — the 'secret death' described by Tertullian[19].

Forceps of varying lengths, with straight or curved blades, were used by physicians; some could be locked into the closed position by a ring (*cyathiscus*) or a dentate clamp. The grasping ends were smooth, dentated or ridged so tissues could be held (*myzon*) or manipulated (*vulsella*) without injury. Forceps were most commonly used to extract missiles and foreign bodies, but some were designed to hold tissues during wound repair and to clamp arteries. Such a clamping instrument was found at Silchester[20]. Opening closed forceps under a surgical incision could expand the size of an operative field without increasing the size of the wound; forceps were also used in this way to increase the drainage of pus from abscesses and boils. Some forceps, such as the *vulsella*, were designed for epilation of turned-in eyelashes of trachoma to prevent corneal abrasion, scarring and blindness; others, such as *staphylagra*, were designed to grasp and crush enlarged haemorrhoids, an infected uvula or other protuberant lesions of the mucous membranes. They also possessed surgical scissors (*forceps excisoria*).

The blades of their scalpels (*scalpelli*) were either fixed or detachable and a few were forged from high-quality Noricum steel. These did not bend or break and could be maintained razor-sharp[21]. Some scalpel blades had a fine point which helped in delicate dissection, while others possessed shapes that were concave, convex or hooked to improve the accuracy of cutting in a variety of different anatomical scenarios.

Blunt hooks (*hamus retusus*), such as the one found at South Shields, were used for dissecting and raising delicate blood vessels, nerves or tendons; sharp hooks (*hamus acutus*), for example the one found at Housesteads, were used for removing tonsils or foreign bodies[22]. These, along with special forceps, were also used to assist in foetus delivery at the time of a catastrophic obstetrical complication, as documented by the bones of an embryotomy found at Poundbury, Dorset[23].

Unobstructed vision of their operative fields was obtained by the use of surgical retractors and tissue forceps with hooks. Bleeding was controlled by local pressure, astringents such as iron rust, tourniquets and ligatures; sometimes, cautery using special instruments (*ferrum candens*) controlled excessive bleeding.

Physicians treated head injuries and some headaches by making holes in the skull (trephination). For this they improved the ancient technique of scraping away the skull bone by developing a trephine drill (*terebra*) or a crown drill (*modiolus*). These were rotated by a thong tied tightly around the shaft, or by a thong attached to a bow or cross-beam. Such instruments allowed better control of the cutting edge against the skull bone and resulted in fewer catastrophic neurological complications. A *meningophylax* was devised to protect the linings of the brain (dura mater and meninges) from injury when bone fragments were removed from the 'burr-hole'. An example of treatment using a *modiolus* was found at York, England[24] and an excellent example of successful trephination for treatment of a depressed fracture of the temporal bone came from Cirencester, England[25]. Before electrically powered bone-drills were developed, neurosurgeons of the late 19th century could have treated neurosurgical emergencies with 'burr-holes' equally as well with the instruments of the *medici*!

These early physicians devised a bivalve speculum used to improve visualization of the operative field with rectal surgery and gynaecological examinations. The most sophisticated medical instrument of ancient times was a bronze 'quadrivalve' speculum, designed to dilate the vagina to visualize the cervix. The penetrating portion of the instrument was shaped like an erect penis (*priapiscus*) which was divided into four quadrants (blades). Each of the sections was connected via levers and hinges to a centrally threaded turn-buckle, and tightening of the screw gradually expanded the blades for controlled, gentle dilatation of the vagina, allowing the operator to view and examine the cervix. The practitioner overcame the problem of a short vagina by using compresses to insulate the labia from the protruding blades of the *priapiscus*[13]. The only improvement in the design of today's vaginal speculum is the use of stainless steel and the availability of different sizes of speculum.

As early as the first century AD, physicians developed hollow bronze tubes (catheters) for emptying the bladder. Separate catheters were designed for the different male and female anatomy. Female catheters were short and slightly curved towards the end; male catheters were longer and S-shaped — one found at Corbridge shows the curved end used to facilitate passage through the upward bend of the posterior urethra where it passes through the prostate gland. (Modern catheters are made from flexible materials which facilitate more comfortable usage.) Retention of urine due to stones and bladder disease (strangury) was a common and painful problem; even the priests of Asclepius could not relieve this by nootherapy alone! Lithotomy instruments were designed for crushing bladder stones, but the dangers of this procedure were such that the oath of Hippocrates cautioned: 'I will not use the knife on sufferers from stone, but will give place to such as are craftsmen therein'.

An experienced eye surgeon used a specially shaped knife with a handle made of bronze, bone or ivory to dislodge the opaque lens (cataract) from in front of the retina. This procedure (called couching) instantly restored sight, with the dislocated lens falling to rest at the bottom of the globe of the eye (coucher). A purpose-designed fine, hollow needle with a protective cover was used to aspirate the lens[18]. The availability of this delicate operation was not restricted to specialized centres; cataract needles have been recovered at Roman forts such as those along Hadrian's Wall at Corbridge and Carlisle.

Physicians used special amputation saws (serrula) which allowed rapid removal of a limb with optimal preservation of residual tissues to facilitate healing. Postoperative rehabilitation programmes incorporated prostheses, including artificial legs made from bronze. A variety of wooden splints and traction apparatus existed for setting and immobilizing fractures and dislocated joints.

Rudimentary syringes and enemas used an inflatable animal bladder for the fluid-containing bag; these instruments featured custom-tailored tips for painless insertion into body orifices in order to douche the vagina, irrigate the bladder, syringe the ears or administer an enema. Wounds were treated by sewing with a needle (acus) and they had discovered that gut could be used as a dissolving suture.

Instruments were boiled or heated between patients' use and efforts were made to prevent cross-infections. The medici had rudimentary knowledge of antisepsis and were skilled in the treatment of wounds, which they washed with vinegar or wine (red preferred). Infected wounds were cleansed with arsenic trioxide (auripigmentum) and arsenic dioxide (sandarica)[26,27], both of which were used as antibacterial agents until the modern antibiotic era. These compounds are extremely toxic and it remains unknown as to whether or not the medici recognized this and avoided arsenic poisoning. They also used tannin to produce a coagulum on the surface of a burn, a practice which continued until the 20th century. Mild infections were treated with topical honey, now known to possess bactericidal properties.

Several other compounds with rubefacient and antiseptic properties aided the treatment of wound infections by creating an additional inflammatory response. This involved an outpouring of white blood cells which removed the infecting organisms. Some of their compounds, such as pitch (resina pinea) and turpentine (resina terebinthina), appeared in pre-antibiotic era pharmacopoeiae with similar Latin names (unguentum picis pini and linimentum terebinthinae)[26]. They treated granulation tissue and ulcers with copper compounds and used a styptic named 'barbarum', similar to the crystals of copper fused with alum that continued to be used empirically by physicians until after World War Two!

They had learnt the value of the counter-irritation produced by poultices and plasters used to treat pleurisy and abscesses. They were skilled at dressing wounds with linen and lint. A specially trained *capsularius* (named after his bandage box) accompanied each fighting unit of the Roman army into battle. Their basic techniques of bandaging (without the benefit of adhesive tape) have continued to present-day.

Although pain was controlled more by restraint than by skilful use of analgesics, myrrh and poppy juice (opium) were administered. The latter was combined with the leaves of henbane and mandrake, both of which contain hyoscyamine (atropine — an antispasmodic)[27,28] and scopolamine (a sedative). These medications, still used by today's anaesthetists, were administered orally and a maintenance level of analgesia was attempted by placing sponges soaked with medication in the patient's mouth.

Cautery was used for both routine and radical treatment. It was used routinely to stop bleeding or to treat varicose veins — these uses did not fit into Hippocrates' treatment of 'last resort' which included malignant tumours and uncontrolled infections. The cautery instrument (*ferrum candens*) was made in different lengths and the treatment ends, used for actual burning, varied in width and shape. A set of four were among the hoard of surgical instruments found at Cramond on the Firth of Forth just west of Edinburgh, Scotland. This hoard, to date the most northerly found in the Roman empire, is housed in the National Museum of Antiquities in Scotland. The treatment ends of the four cauteries range from a fine point, through narrow curve and broad curve, to a spatula shape 2 cm diameter and 1 mm thick[29] (Figure 68).

In 1996, the first definite and properly excavated ancient British medical kit was found at Stanway, near Colchester. The *instrumentarium* contained a complete set of 13 basic tools of ancient surgery: scalpels, sharp and blunt hooks, spring forceps, handled needles, a scoop probe and a surgical saw. Ralph Jackson, of the British Museum, dated the burial to 50–60 AD. He described it as 'not only the earliest identifiable kit from Britain but one of the earliest surviving *instrumentaria* from anywhere in the ancient world'. 'The basic surgical kit' was described in *The Hippocratic corpus* and a physician was advised to keep it with him at all times. Jackson concluded that: 'There is no doubt that the healer who used the Stanway *instrumentarium* was in contact with Roman practitioners, and was probably versed in the precepts of classical medicine'[30].

Physicians carried compact *instrumentaria* allowing them to undertake 'minor surgery' at the patient's home or on the spot. Elective or major surgery was performed at the 'office' or 'clinic', which had facilities for operating in good light and where medical students or apprentices served as surgical assistants (internes or house surgeons), performing duties such as keeping the patient steady and holding a retractor or sponge. The 'clinics' also had facilities for 'sterilizing' instruments and for cautery.

Status of the early physician
The status of early Greek and Roman physicians varied over the 700 years of Asclepius' predominant role as god of medicine. The academic and social upper classes of the Greek and Roman world considered manual labour and the practice of medicine beneath their dignity. In addition to class distinction, snobbery and patronage, diverse demographical factors influenced the physician's place in Greek and Roman society. In order to estimate the status of an individual physician, the following questions had to be answered.

Was he a native in the subject country or an immigrant? What did the native population think of foreigners? For example, in the third century BC, Greeks were suspect in Rome but by the second century AD, Greek-trained physicians were considered the best in the ancient world.

The social background and caste of the doctor also influenced his status. Was he a slave in Greece or a postconquest slave in Rome? Was he a slave employed by the social elite or one who worked for civic government? Were his patients slaves, society damsels or political leaders? Was he a freedman or a citizen? Was he a *medicus ordinarius* in the Roman army or a private physician to the commandant? What was his training? Was he a self-professed healer or a charlatan? Was he a professional who had trained via the apprentice system? Did he belong to a 'guild' or collegium? Was he trained at a medical school? Did he have a broad education including philosophy? Did he train at Cos, Alexandria, Pergamum or one of the other sparse academic facilities for teaching medicine? Was he a Hippocratic or non-Hippocratic professional?

Their status was also influenced by their ability to debate, denigrate and one-up the diagnosis, prognosis and treatment of fellow practitioners. Patients of high social and financial status had an entourage of physicians from diverse disciplines; this custom continues today among the wealthy who often have one or two specialists attending to each of their complaints. Among this assemblage, physicians were not discrete in their competitiveness; they were immodest in their self-aggrandizement and ridiculed their colleagues' mistakes in public. For example, Antonius Musa gained fame by serendipity while Galen enjoyed the 'gamesmanship' of medical practice but his successes were based on superior knowledge and ability. Both physicians gained the ultimate rung of the status ladder by becoming physician to the emperor and by reaping great financial rewards.

A complete discussion of the effects of demographics on the status of early doctors is beyond the scope of this book, but all the various pieces of information are tied together by two common facts: first, even the Caesars stood naked before the physician and, second, Asclepius was the god of medicine worshipped by all practitioners.

The qualifications of healers in the classical world differed widely. Those at the top had been trained professionally under the apprentice-ship system or rarely at the medical schools of Cos, Alexandria, Pergamum, Cnidus and Croton; those at the bottom were the self-professed healers and charlatans. Although the apprenticeship system was biased towards nepotism, others did enter the profession but family favouritism might explain the entry of women into this male-dominated profession. Standards of training would have developed for each locale and some apprentices might have been exposed to Hippocratic writings and thereby influenced to attain higher standards. When medical practitioners became more numerous in ancient Greece, methods of practice expanded. Some continued as itinerant physicians while others congregated at Asclepian temple sites. Some preferred the security of being employed by wealthy families or local municipalities. Despite their apprenticeship training and formation of medical guilds, most doctors in ancient Greece remained low on the social scale and were equated to tradesmen.

After the conquest of Greece by Rome, many doctors became slaves owned by prominent families or worked under the republic. Eventually, some slaves were able to improve their status by buying their freedom and becoming a 'freedman'. A few of these acquired powerful patrons who were able to influence the emperor to grant citizenship to themselves and their families[31]. Some slave doctors entered the service of the Roman army and, after their term of duty, gained a grant of land and citizenship. Extraordinary physicians became society doctors, teachers, writers or senior medical officers in the Roman army. In later centuries, Greek physicians were regarded as the best in the world and it became necessary for doctors to have had Greek training to attain status. In recent times, there was a similar concept in the British Empire where doctors from colonial countries enhanced their status at home by taking postgraduate training at London or Edinburgh. This training was proudly proclaimed in their homelands, and even those who failed the British examinations placed 'MRCP London (failed)' on their office doors and stationery.

In ancient Rome, there were laws which facilitated quack physicians and charlatans as all that was needed to practice medicine was an affidavit or '*professio*' where one professed that he was a healer. The *professores* of medicine contrasted sharply with the professionals who had undergone some type of formal training. However, Scribonius Largus noted ironically that a few of those without formal training provided better care than those professionally trained! The incompetents from each group became subject matter for the sport of the satirists.

The duration of medical training is not known but it varied between the extremes of very short and very long. Jackson recorded two *medici ocularii* from the army who died in Rome at the ages of 17 and 19 years. The tombstone of the *medicus ordinarius* Anicius Ingenuus, found at the hospital site of the fort at Housesteads on Hadrian's Wall, recorded his death at the age of 25 years. Galen completed 12 years study to build the foundations of his career as specialist, author and master clinician.

The professionals were divided into two categories: Hippocratic and non-Hippocratic. After the death of Hippocrates, groups of physicians, teachers and philosophers split from the Hippocratic doctrines and formed separate medical systems[32]. These were spawned in Alexandria but grew and flourished in Rome. The groups were composed of important practitioners of the time who made many significant contributions to medical advances.

Plato led the *Pragmatists* who accepted the theory of the four humours; subjective philosophy, however, replaced clinical observation and objectivity. *Empiricism* concerned itself with the effects of treatment but not causes. Their opinions were based on clinical experience, observation and prognosis.

Methodism evolved from the first century BC practice of Asclepiades (who was not related to the god but his name favoured his career and his school adopted the name 'Asclepiads'). He was of low social status and worked as a miller to pay for his tuition. Asclepiades studied rhetoric at Athens and presumably medicine at Alexandria. In 91 BC, he came to Rome where his personal magnetism, rhetoric and gentle treatments made him the most popular doctor in the city. He deliberately abandoned the humoral theory and believed that the physician, not nature, cured disease. He regarded the healthy body as being composed of moving atoms or corpuscles of varying size, which were imperceptible to the senses and flowed continuously in fluids through body pores. Disease resulted when the atomic motion and flow was altered. Bathing was an essential component of therapy. His most enduring success was the development of a tracheotomy (making a hole in the airway tube) to relieve obstructed breathing.

Themison, a student of Asclepiades, developed his atomic theories further with the doctrine of *Methodism* and added that the moving atoms also needed to move through body pores which were in a state of relaxation or contraction. He related disease to contraction and relaxation of body pores as judged by evacuations, secretions and fever. Their system of therapeutics opened pores by rigorous diet, warm baths, poultices, humid air, bleeding and medicines, while pores were closed by cold baths, air and styptics. Antonius Musa, a freedman of Greek descent, was a Methodist who gained wealth and fame. He prescribed cold baths and lettuce to cure Emperor Augustus' abdominal pain. The cause had been considered a liver abscess and the conventional therapy was heat; however, Musa obtained dramatic results with the use of cold baths and compresses[33]. This treatment may have serendipitously treated intestinal typhoid and its modern counterpart was the similar treatment given to the Prince of Wales in 1871[34]. Musa was rewarded handsomely by the emperor who honoured him with gold, immunity from taxes and the commissioning of a sculpture portraying him in the guise of Aesculapius. The completed statue was placed beside a similar official statue of the god. A modern clinical assessment of Methodism raises the question as to whether or not the insensible atoms of varying sizes were in fact red and white blood corpuscles that are invisible to the eye and can only be seen using a microscope and special staining. As a corollary to the corpuscle question, did the pores refer only to sweat pores in the skin or did they include minute blood vessels (capillaries) and the entire vascular system? The state of blood corpuscles and size of blood vessels are the essentials of haematological and cardiovascular diseases.

Pneumatism was another system using *pneuma* (a spirit or breath) that entered the body by breathing, was distributed throughout the body via the left side of the heart and arteries, and reacted with warmth and moisture.

Eclecticism adhered to no single system but took ideas according to any source to explain and treat illness. Galen was an eclectic and embraced all five theories as well as being a believer in the powers of Aesculapius. Modern medicine is truly eclectic as today it embraces a multitude of ever-increasing new, diverse scientific disciplines.

Physicians with a specialty

Most doctors were general practitioners but, as happens in present-day, isolated medical practices resulted in the acquisition of varying degrees of specialization. This is a consequence of individual doctors' likes and dislikes, as well as the availability of expert opinion. For example, in some busy general practices one doctor may be interested in obstetrics while another may not; this frequently leads to fellow physicians referring all their deliveries to a colleague who, over a period of time, gradually becomes more experienced and skilled in delivering babies. Similarly, a doctor who dislikes obstetrics may enjoy treating patients with skin rashes and, with time, he too gains more experience in dermatology such that his colleagues begin to refer their patients with skin problems to him. In rural areas of the world, where there is an absence of specialists, general physicians may become anaesthetists, surgeons, fracture specialists and surgical assistants. In the Roman army, even the *capsularii* and *medicii ordinarii* became experts at removing embedded missiles.

Inventive doctors designed their own specialized instruments; these simplified the performance of difficult procedures and facilitated the development of specialized practitioners. Some Asclepiads and *medici* had more extensive experience with eye disease, bone setting, haemorrhoids, fissures, tonsils, dentistry, and locomotor disorders.

Eye diseases were common in the ancient world and '*medici ocularii*' was a term used by some to describe their skills. These 'specialists' operated on cataracts by couching and used special scalpels and needles for lens removal. They also had special instruments to facilitate surgery on the eyelid. Several effective ointments and salves were available for treating a variety of common eye diseases. There is an interesting historical record for these because, for convenience, the ingredients of their various preparations were hardened with gums and made into a solid stick (*collyrium*). These were circumscribed with the names of the medical practitioner and his special medicine: the medical formula and the disease for which it was prescribed.

This complicated inscription was simplified by the use of special oculist's stamps made from steatite or greenish schist. These were square with an inscription on each of the four edges. The letters were cut in intaglio form and written from right to left so that, when stamped on the *collyrium*, they made an impression which read from left to right. Two hundred and ninety-six specimens of stone stamp have been found, mainly from north-western Europe; 28 of these were discovered in Britain and one in Eire. The British examples relate to 29 salves for 12 ailments ranging from scars to running eyes[35].

Surgeons became specialized in other areas, especially for complicated fractures, trephination of the skull and for those who could perform some types of plastic surgery. Today's plastic surgeons perform elective cosmetic surgery for wrinkles, prominent noses and small or sagging breasts but their ancient predecessors removed the branding scars of slaves or produced an artificial prepuce to conceal the ritual circumcision of the Jews[36].

Soranus was an outstanding second century gynaecologist who practised according to the Methodist school. Their concept that illness was caused by an imbalance of closed or open pores can be translated into obstetrical and gynaecological practice. The relaxation and contraction of the uterus and relaxation (dilatation) of the birth canal are the basic physiology of pregnancy and many gynaecological conditions. It remains unknown as to whether or not Soranus became interested in his specialty due to his Methodist training or if obstetrical problems attracted him to their regimens. He wrote surprisingly modern texts describing obstetrical and gynaecological practice[37] and described treatment for morning sickness, dysmenorrhoea and pica (the rare manifestation of iron deficiency involving a craving for a variety of non-dietary substances) [personal communication: Dr Lindsay Allason-Jones, University of Newcastle]. Midwives managed most deliveries but physicians were consulted on difficult labours. For these, he described manual traction, the use of hooks and forceps. His recommendations for swaddling an infant have been found at York and the only example to date of his method of embryotomy was found at Poundbury, Dorset[38].

Medicae (female doctors) frequently specialized in the treatment of women's diseases and were accepted by Roman society as a whole. Furthermore, a statement included in a finely inscribed dedication found at Lyons attests to their financial success: '*de sua pecunia dedit*' (gave with her own money)[39].

Specialists were not uniformly available but congregated in the larger cities such as Alexandria and Rome, where there were adequate pools of patients to sustain a lucrative practice.

Medical fees

Ancient physicians practised medicine in order to earn a living. Their fees were not low and it was only later that a form of a public medical service evolved. Treatment of the poor was at the discretion of the individual physician, but most were probably like Galen who prided himself on 'treating senators and slaves with the same scrupulousness'; this altruism was balanced by the wealth and fame bestowed on him by the social elite. Before the advent of socialized medicine, a similar system of balanced billing and equally scrupulous medical care was in effect in clinics and on public wards of general hospitals in Canada, Britain, the US and other countries.

Summary

Many artefacts associated with the medical practice of the Greek and Roman physicians have survived. There are also numerous ancient medical texts, including the encyclopaedic work of Celsus (born c25 BC) which described contemporary dietary therapy, pharmacology and surgical techniques[34]. Reading the work of ancient authors results in a sense of amazement at their knowledge of medical treatment.

Asclepiads and *medici* applied the principles of conservative therapy and knew the value of 'tincture of time' (see chapter 5). They tried to balance body humours by cupping, purging, clystering, administering emetics and strict dietary regimens. Their medicines were dispensed as tablets, powders, snuff, mixtures, lotions and balms. Instruments that resembled modern day counterparts were developed which facilitated their performance of many surgical procedures. They also possessed the true art of medicine — the intuitive ability to make the patient feel better despite the difficulties of his illness and the limitations of available therapy.

The status of ancient physicians varied as did their competence and training. The hypothetical lowest would have been a Hebrew slave from Greece who had been taken to Rome to treat slaves working at the cattle market. Musa was at the other end of the spectrum; by serendipity, he cured Augustus of typhoid and attained the heights of success and wealth. Galen, using his skills and competence, became the eternal icon of Roman medical practice.

Unfortunately, the availability of exemplary services in the ancient world was sporadic and, unlike today, their local deficiencies could not be compensated by air ambulance and telemedicine.

Notes and references

1. Edelstein EJ, Edelstein L. *Asclepius, a collection and interpretation of the testimonies. Volume 2*. Baltimore: Johns Hopkins Press, 1945: 139.
2. Toole H. *Asclepius, Part 1: Asclepius in history and legend*. St Louis: CV Mosby Company, 1963: Surgery vol 53-3: 387–400.
3. Toole H. *Asclepius, Part II: Critical analysis of the cures attributed to Asclepius*. St Louis: CV Mosby Company, 1963: Surgery vol 53-3: 401–19.
4. Goold GP, ed. *Hippocrates Vols I, II, IV*. Translated by Jones WHJ. Loeb Classical Library. Massachusetts: Harvard University Press and London: William Heinemann Ltd. Reprinted: Vol I 1984, Vol II 1992, Vol IV 1992.

5. Goold GP, ed. *Hippocrates Vols V, VI*. Translated by Potter P. Loeb Classical Library. Massachusetts: Harvard University Press and London: William Heinemann Ltd, 1958.

6. There is ethnic variation in natural immunity; this has played a significant role in world history. The native Mexicans had no natural immunity to smallpox which the Spanish invaders brought to Mexico. Similarly, the native people of the Pacific Islands were decimated by measles which the British explorers brought. In Canada, the arctic Eskimos have increased susceptibility to tuberculosis.

7. For Greek text see: Goold GP, ed. *Hippocrates Vol IV*. Loeb Classical Library. Massachusetts: Harvard University Press and London: William Heinemann Ltd, 1987.

8. The four elements of Empedocles were associated with the physical world, the body, the seasons and personality. It was believed that a balance of these controlled health and temperament: a) fire was associated with: hot, rough, red blood; spring; choleric temperament; b) water was associated with: cold, smooth, white phlegm; winter; phlegmatic temperament; c) air was associated with: dry, salt, sweet, black bile; autumn; melancholic temperament; and d) earth was associated with: moist, acid, yellow bile; summer; sanguineous temperament. Quoted from Celsus *de Medicina*, translated by Spencer WG. Massachusetts: Harvard University Press and London: William Heinemann Ltd, 1960.

9. Schouten J. *The rod and serpent of Asklepios*. New York: Elsevier Publishing Company, 1967: 47. According to Dr Schouten, a Dutch art historian, Telesphorus was associated with the trochar for bloodletting; this is not a clinical interpretation of his associated role. Incisions over the vein were the method of initiating blood flow. Although there were no trochars in the modern sense in the instrumentation of Greek physicians, Schouten describes the cupping vessel as a trochar. If Telesphorus were associated with the procedure of wet cupping (venesection) then he would be eligible to become god of modern day haematologists!

10. The Lilac Gardens at the Royal Botanic Gardens, Kew, London, has a descriptive plaque describing lilacs as 'belonging to the genus *Syringa*, whose scientific name comes from the Greek word Syrinx, meaning a pipe, referring to the hollow stem — a characteristic of lilacs. Doctors in ancient Greece used the stems to inject medicine.' The ancient syringe was half plant stem and half bladder. A firm plant stem could have served as an ancient trochar, as could the quill of bird feathers.

11. Brock AJ. *Galen on the natural faculties*. Massachusetts: Harvard University Press and London: William Heinemann Ltd, 1952.

12. Bender GA. *Great moments in pharmacy*. Detroit: Northwood Institute Press, 1966: 32-5, 40–3.

13. Jackson R. *Doctors and diseases in the Roman empire*. London: British Museum Press, 1988: 82.

14. (a) Bidwell PT. *Britannia* XVII 1986; **449**: no 77, item 54.

    (b) Guido M. *The healing hand man and wound healing in the ancient world*. Massachusetts: Harvard University Press, 1975: 186–8. This describes the Greeks as using wine to cleanse wounds with bacteriostatic action resulting from a polyphenol (malvoside). In addition, wine per se rather than its alcohol content has a bacteriocidal action. This effect is transient because body proteins bind the active principles rapidly.

15. Hamilton JS. Scribonius Largus on the medical profession. *Bull Hist Med* 1986; **60**: 209–16.

16. The Frisians, who gave medicine to the Romans, called dock 'britannica'. The scientific names are *Radix britannica* and the Elder Pliny's *Rumex augustifolius* or *Rumex obtusifolius*. Remains of it have been found in the Romano-British towns of Caerwent, Carmarthen and Southwark. Dock still grows wild in Britain, especially in areas where there are large numbers of stinging nettles. Folklore recommends it for the relief of the histamine weal from stinging nettles — and it works!

17. The Roman denarius was used as a unit of weight. Initially in 187 BC, the denarius weighed 4 scruples (80 grains) of pure silver but underwent a series of debasements of both weight and silver content throughout Roman history. During Augustus' reign (27 BC–14 AD), the coin weighed 61.64 grains. In 58 AD, Scribonius Largus demonstrated his bias to Rome by commenting that 84 denarii made a pound and to ignore the number of Greek drachmae that made up this unit of weight. Shortly after this comment, the denarius of Nero (54–68 AD) was reduced to 52.65 grains and the bronze aes of Roman currency, which began at 10 ounces, was gradually reduced to 2 ounces. Each debasement of coinage created a domino effect ending with the scrupulus equating to 1/288th of an aes and was the smallest unit of Roman weight. These changes complicated the dispensing of prescriptions, such as the one described by the Elder Pliny. There was probably a good market for the original coins and the Asclepiads and the Chironidae (pharmacists) became the first coin collectors. The scruple (20 grains) was still used as an apothecary weight until the international acceptance of the metric system; the changes in weight of Roman coins made the physician's problems with the recent conversion from apothecary weights to the metric system seem like child's play.

18. Gilson AG. A group of surgical and medical instruments from Corbridge. *Sonderdruck aus dem Saalburg-Jahrbuch* XXXVII. Berlin: Verlag Walter de Gruyter, 1981. Gilson described the largest group of Roman surgical instruments found in Britain to date.

19. Wells C. A Roman surgical instrument from Norfolk. *Antiquity* 1967; 4: 139–41.

20. Boon GC. *The Roman town of Calleva*. London: David and Charles, Newton Abbot, 1974. Finds at this site include: a pair of artery forceps, specimens of sandarac (disulphide of arsenic), St John's wort and henbane (*Hyoscyamus niger*).

21. Jackson R. *Doctors and diseases in the Roman empire*. London: British Museum Press, 1988: 114.

22. Allason-Jones L. Two unrecognised surgical instruments. In: *Archaeologia Aeliana*, 5 VII, Museum notes, 1979.

23. Farwell DE, Molleson TI. *Poundbury: volume 2 the cemeteries*. Dorset Natural History and Archaeological Society, 1993: no 11.

24. Brothwell DR. Osteological evidence of the use of a surgical modiolus in a Romano-British population. An aspect of primitive technology. *J Arch Sci* 1974; 1: 209–17.

25. Wells C. Une curieuse blessure un squelette du deuxieme siecle AD. *Trav Doc du Center de Paleopathologie* 1977; 4: 9–13. (Also in McWhirr A, Viner L, Wells C. Romano-British cemeteries at Cirencester. In: *The human burials Cirencester excavations II*. Cirencester Excavation Committee, 1982.)

26. Ferguson JKW, Lucas GHW. *Materia medica*. Toronto: University of Toronto Press, 1948.

27. Richmond IA. The Roman army medical service. *Medical Gazette* (Durham University) 1952; **46**(3): 2–6.

28. Poppy seeds have been found at Carlisle, and henbane seeds at Silchester and Carmarthen. Allason-Jones L. *Health care in the Roman north, medicine in Northumbria*. Newcastle-upon-Tyne: The Pybus Society for the History and Bibliography of Medicine, 1993.

29. Gilson GG. A group of Roman surgical and medical instruments from Cramond, Scotland. *Medizin Historisches Journal* 1983; **18**: 4.

30. Dr Philip Crummy, director of the Colchester Archaeological Trust, stated the instruments indicate that an exchange of medical knowledge took place in the early years of the invasion. He noted this individual represents the earliest known doctor in England. (Crummy P. The Stanway Burials. *Curr Archaeol* 1997; **153**: 337–42.) Ralph Jackson, the authority on medical instruments in Roman Britain, described these finds under the title: Jackson R. An ancient British medical kit from Stanway, Essex. *Lancet* 1997; **350**: 1471–3. Jackson has also written the following papers of significance: The composition of Roman medical *instrumentaria* as an indicator of medical practice: a provisional assessment. In: van der Eijk Ph J, Horstmannshoff, HFJ, Schrijvers PH, eds. Ancient medicine in its socio-cultural context. Papers read at the congress held at Leiden University, 13–15 April 1992. Amsterdam/Atlanta GA: *Clio Medica* 1995; **1**: 189–207. Jackson R. A set of Roman medical instruments from Italy. *Britannia* 1986; **17**: 119–67.

31. Mattern SP. Physicians and the Roman imperial aristocracy: the patronage of therapeutics. *The American Association for the History of Medicine*, no 1, Spring 1999.

32. Lyons AS, Petrucelli RJ. *Medicine an illustrated history*. New York: Henry N Abrams Inc Publishers, 1978.

33. In 23 BC, Musa also prescribed the same treatment for the inflamed eyes of the Roman poet Horace. The writer complained that his taking of cold baths made him unpopular at the fashionable hot spring resort of Baiae. Horace recorded that the cold baths were located at fontes Clusini (near modern Chiusi, north of Rome). In 1992, the Guila Paolucci of the local museum and, in 1994, the University of Arizona excavated at nearby Chianciano and located the largest ancient spa pool in Italy. The excavators, Soren and Romer, concluded that this was the site of Horace's healing spring. It is more than a coincidence that each year, thousands of people still visit Chianciano to take the local waters and baths for treatment of liver and stomach conditions! Soren D, Romer F. Horace's healing spring. *Archaeology* 1999; **52**: 47–8.

34. Celsus (born c25 BC) described the 'art of medicine' as being divided into three parts: 'one being that which cures through diet, another through medicaments, and the third by hand'. The text from the eight volumes of his *de Medicina* has survived and modern translations give a catalogue of dietary therapy, pharmacology and surgery contemporary with the beginning of the first century AD. It remains unknown whether or not Celsus was a physician, but his works are consistent with those of a science-writer and an encyclopaedist than reflecting the style of one who has treated a dying patient or who has experienced the unpleasantness of vomitus or rectal examinations. Celsus *de Medicina*, translated by Spencer WG in three volumes, Massachusetts: Harvard University Press and William Heinemann Ltd, 1960. Spencer's introduction to volume 2 and 9 referred to the Prince of Wales's attack of typhoid which was treated by cold packs.

35. Jackson R. A new collyrium stamp from Cambridge and a corrected reading of the stamp from Caistor-by-Norwich. *Britannia* 1990; **21**: 275–83.

36. Jackson R. *Doctors and diseases in the Roman empire*. London: British Museum Press, 1988: 123–4.

37. English translations of gynaecology by Soranus are rare. Soranus had no faith in the tradition of amulets and charms as an adjunct to a safe delivery.
38. Farwell DE, Molleson TL. *Excavations at Poundbury 1966–80. Vol II: the Cemeteries*. Dorset Natural History and Archaeological Society, 1993: no 11.
39. In recent times, women were unable to gain entry to medical school until the latter half of the 19th century. Elizabeth Blackwell was the first female doctor of modern times. She entered the Geneva Medical School of Western New York disguised as a man and graduated in 1849. Even after graduation, women were not accepted as 'real doctors'. As late as the 1940s, a female general practitioner was not accepted in the Dorset town of Beaminster, England. In Canada in 1971, the Royal College of Physicians and Surgeons were sending invitations to their convocation ceremony addressed 'You and your wife are invited to attend...'. My colleague in practice was a *medica* and asked, 'What do I do? I do not have a wife!'

Chapter 9

Asclepius everywhere

Asclepius was worshipped throughout the Graeco-Roman world and became one of the most important deities of classical antiquity. This chapter reviews the evidence for this statement and corroborates the words of Apuleius, a second century AD Roman writer, sometimes referred to as a 'platonic philosopher' who wrote: 'Aesculapius ubique' (Aesculapius everywhere) — *De Deo Socratis* XV 153 (ET 254).

The cult of Asklepios, written by Alice Walton, contains a chapter entitled 'Index to locality of cults'[1]. This lists geographically 368 Asclepieia located by archaeological, literary, epigraphic and numismatic sources (Table 2, see Appendix 3; Map 1 indicates the location of these sites). One hundred and sixty-five of these locations are known only by coins bearing one or more of the types of Asclepius, Hygieia or Telesphorus (Table 3, see Appendix 3). Walton's conclusion about the number of Asclepieia is overstated as she accepted an isolated dedication to Asclepius as sufficient evidence for identification of a temple site whereas an altar, statue or an inscription indicates a devotee and a place of worship but not an Asclepieion. Despite this criticism, her review remains the primary reference for the locations of Asclepian worship and is a strong foundation on which additional evidence can be built. The format of the updated review presented here follows the Walton 'geographical sequence' to simplify comparison by future reviewers. New additions use modern place names and, when available, the Latin name, but Walton's original use of the Greek κ for C and her other minor linguistic differences are preserved. Alice Walton excluded 'the Latin writers' from this chapter and, like the Edelsteins, did not include some Latin inscriptions. These decisions result in the omission of locations in Britain, Gaul, Spain and elsewhere in the Roman empire.

Additional sites of Aesculapius, Salus or Telesphorus worship in Roman Britain

There are 13 sites of worship associated with Aesculapius or Salus in Roman Britain that were not listed by Walton (Table 4). All but two of these additional locations are sites at or near a Roman fort and were probably associated with physicians, four of whom made their

Map 1   The ancient world in Roman times

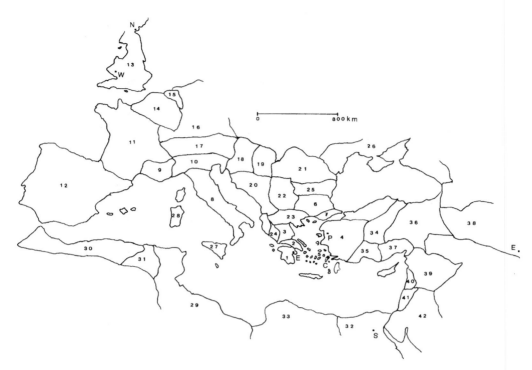

Drawn by C Buhle

Numbers indicate ancient name and brackets indicate modern region

1. Peloponnesus (southern Greece; E = location of Epidaurus)
2. Attica
3. Thessaly (eastern peninsula of central Greece)
4. Asia (western part of Asia Minor which included Mysia, Lydia, Caria, Phrygia, Troas & Ionia); P = the site of Pergamum
5. Aegean Islands and Doric Islands; C = island of Cos
6. Thracia (central & south Bulgaria)
7. Pontus (north-east Turkey)
8. Italia (Italy)
9. G Narbonensis (Provence region of France)
10. G Cisalpina (north Italy)
11. Gallia (France)
12. Hispania (Spain & Portugal)
13. Britannia (England, Wales, parts of Scotland)
14. Belgica (Belgium)
15. Germania Inferior (northern Germany)
16. Germania Superior (southern Germany)
17. Alpes & Noricum (Switzerland, Austria & parts of neighbours)
18. Pannonia Superior (western parts of Hungary & former Yugoslavia)
19. Pannonia Inferior (eastern parts of Hungary & former Yugoslavia)
20. Dalmatia (Adriatic coast of former Yugoslavia)
21. Dacia (Romania)
22. Moesia Superior (Serbia)
23. Macedonia (northern Greece)

24. Epirus (north-west Greece)
25. Moesia Inferior (north Bulgaria)
26. North of Black Sea (southern Ukraine & east Georgia)
27. Sicilia (Sicily)
28. Sardinia (Sardinia)
29. Africa (province which included Algeria, Libya, Cyrenaica, Mauretania & Egypt)
30. Mauretania (Morocco & part of Algeria)
31. Numidia (Algeria)
32. Aegyptus (Egypt)
33. Cyrenaica (eastern Libya)
34. Galatia (central Turkey)
35. Lycia & Pamphylia (southern Turkey)
36. Cappadocia (eastern Turkey)
37. Cilicia (southern Turkey)
38. Media (western Iran)
39. Syria (Syria)
40. Phoenicia (Lebanon)
41. Judea (Israel)
42. Arabia (north-western Arabia)

W = Brecon, the westernmost evidence for Asclepius
N = Carpow, the northernmost evidence for Asclepius
S = Memphis, the southernmost evidence for Asclepius
E = Ecbatana, the easternmost evidence for Asclepius

inscriptions in Greek (see chapter 7). A fifth example of a Greek background comes from an inscription at Tunstall, Lancashire, where the dedication to Asclepius and Hygieia was written in Latin script but the Roman equivalent, 'Aesculapius and Salus', was omitted (Figure 64)[2].

The inclusion of Birdoswald and Carvoran in Table 4 requires additional comment. A small, weathered relief attributed to Aesculapius and a statue of Telesphorus were found at Birdoswald in the 19th century[3]. It has recently been argued that Mercury, rather than Aesculapius, was depicted here as the serpent-entwined staff was held in the god's left hand [personal communication: Allison-Jones L, 1995]. This is an unwarranted premise because Aesculapius has been depicted on ancient art holding his staff in an ambidextrous fashion. However, the nudity of the god and the possible depiction of two serpents supports a depiction of Mercury but if the small, hooded figure found there is Telesphorus then this is evidence for worship of Aesculapius.

A small, uninscribed altar, depicting a boar on its left side and a serpent on its right, was found at Carvoran (the Roman name being Magnis) on Hadrian's Wall. Reverend J Collingwood Bruce interprets the boar as symbolic of the 20th legion and the serpent of the faith of the donor[4]. The most likely faith represented is that of Aesculapius.

In 1995, the British Museum acquired a bronze figurine of Aesculapius discovered near Chichester, West Sussex (Noviomagus Regnorum). Although small in size (64.1 mm high), it depicts the traditional face, hair and beard of Aesculapius who is clothed in a *himation* and supported by his staff. That it exhibits signs of considerable wear attests to its frequent use as part of a healing ritual (Figure 23)[5].

A bas-relief, which referred to the Asclepian myth, was found 20 feet below present street level at the Cross Street Bath site near the temple of Sulis Minerva, Bath (Aquae Sulis). This depicts Coronis and Apollo accompanied by a serpent and a dog (Figure 22)[6]. The centre of the eastern pediment of the temple of Sulis Minerva featured a Gorgon's head. Although the Gorgon was an attribute of Athena (Minerva), she was also depicted on the throne of Asclepius at Epidaurus. Athena gave Asclepius some of the Gorgon's blood enabling him to revive the dead. Luna, holding a rod associated with a serpent, is portrayed on a pediment of a building on the north side of the temple's principal altar. The lash of her traditional whip was serpent-shaped; in the fifth century AD, Proclus described her association with Aesculapius: 'Porphyrius states that it is reasonable to believe that even the art of

healing comes from Athena, because also Asclepius is a lunar intellect'.
(ET 304)

Two other depictions of serpents have been described at Bath[7].
These may be associated with Minerva's healing role in the Roman
world. She was depicted with Aesculapius on a statue found at
Coventina's Well, Hadrian's Wall (Figure 14) and had the title
'Minerva Medica'. On occasions, Athena was also regarded as Hygieia.
It is likely that Minerva was the healing deity of Aquae Sulis but there
was an association with Aesculapius, especially for the Roman soldiers
who came to Bath to convalesce from illness and injury.

The inscription to Aesculapius from Greenwich (Londinium) (RIB
37) is a debatable addition. This dedication was found at an important
Roman site (possibly a shrine), in Greenwich Park, London, and reads:
'...culap' or '...cular'. 'Culap' represents an inscription to Aesculapius[8,9], but Ralph Jackson reviewed the lettering and felt that the
inscription was definitely 'cular', which would exclude Aesculapius
[personal communication: Jackson R, 1993]. However, there is a
remote possibility that the engraver had some knowledge of Greek and
combined this with muddled thinking. The Greek letter P is written in
Latin text as an R. What if he knew Aesculapius was a Greek god and
thought the P was in fact a Greek rho (P) which should be written in
Latin text as an R?

Undoubtedly, many Roman sites in Britain remain to be identified.
For example, in 1994, a hitherto unknown Roman town was
discovered at Heybridge Pool near Maldon in Essex (*Essex Chronicle*,
1994). In 1995, Dr Vince Gaffney, from the University of
Birmingham, released preliminary results from a geophysical survey
of the Roman town of Viroconium (Wroxeter) that he had
coordinated; this revealed an unexcavated 'British Pompeii' (*London
Times*, 1995). Finds such as these indicate the potential for further
discoveries relating to Aesculapius and Greek-trained physicians,
especially as none of the 'active' *valetudinaria* of the legionary fortresses
in Britain have been fully excavated. If these are found, it is hoped they
will lead to discoveries similar to those at Novae, near Sviston,
Bulgaria, where a building constructed on the ruins of the
valetudinarium of the legionary fortress of the First Italian Legion
contained a dedication to Asclepius and Hygieia. In addition, at
Bingen and Neuss in Germany, excavation of the *valetudinaria* revealed
large numbers of surgical instruments[10–14].

Most British legionary fortresses were constructed at sites that
became Roman towns and then evolved into the centres of modern
cities. However, the fortress built by Vespasian in c44 AD and the

Table 4   13 sites of worship, not listed by Walton, associated with Aesculapius or Salus in Roman Britain

Name	County/country	Roman name
Bath	Avon	Aquae Sulis
Binchester	Durham	Vinovia
Birdoswald (Hadrian's Wall)	Northumberland	Camboglanna
Caerleon	Wales	Isca Silurum
Carvoran	Northumberland	Magnis
Carrowburgh (Coventina's Well)	Northumberland	Broclitia
Chesters (Hadrian's Wall)	Northumberland	Cilurnum
Chichester	West Sussex	Noviomagus Regnorum
Corbridge	Northumberland	Corstopitum
London (Greenwich, possible)	London	Londinium
Overborough (Tunstall)	Lancashire	Galacum
Risingham	Northumberland	Habitancum
South Shields	Durham	Arbeia

Second Augusta Legion at Lake Farm near Wimborne Minster, Dorset, were discovered in 1966[15]. The potential for finding a military hospital at this site is great as the fort was built to facilitate conquest of the many 'impregnable' hillforts of the Durotrigian tribe. The Lake site has not been fully investigated and the report of work to date by Poole Museum awaits publication.

Additional sites of Asclepian worship in the Graeco-Roman world

The findings of these additional locations in Britain led to a comprehensive, but not exhaustive, review of archaeological, historical and numismatic literature from other areas of the Graeco-Roman world. Ninety-six additional sites of Asclepian worship were identified — these are summarized in Table 5 and are detailed in Tables 5a—e.

Table 5   96 sites of Asclepian worship from other sources

Location	Reference	No sites
GAUL, Germany etc	Table 5a	45
EDELSTEIN	Table 5b	21
SPAIN	Table 5c	6
MISCELLANEOUS	Table 5d	12
UNCOLLATED	Table 5e	12 (Coins alone 9)

The boundaries of Roman Gaul included those of present-day France, Belgium, parts of Germany and Switzerland. Walton's review encompassed only a small portion of the province, namely: Gallia Narbonensis (which included parts of southern France), together with Gallia Cisalpina (which included the northern part of present-day Italy)[1]. Many bas-reliefs, statues, busts and inscriptions of various gods have been found in Roman Gaul. These were meticulously catalogued by Esperandieu, who published his findings in a series of 15 volumes[16,17]. Each volume was published separately between 1907 and 1966, and every specimen assigned a number; the first series was reprinted in 1976[16]. Table 5a lists the locations of the 29 additional bas-reliefs, statues and busts of Asclepius (Esculape) and Hygieia (Hygie) listed by Esperandieu; the French names of the sites are listed alphabetically and are followed, where available, by the Latin name. In 1982, Sikora reviewed the occurrence of Asclepius in Roman Gaul and added five inscriptions and four reliefs that were not included by Walton and Esperandieu. These nine additional sites are also listed in Table 5a. Sikora noted that the sites for Aesculapius in Gaul were along main north/south routes and concluded from her findings that they represented greater worship by Romans than by the local inhabitants, who did not accept Aesculapius as their god of medicine[18].

Other studies have revealed seven additional sites in the province not described by Walton. There were two large legionary fortresses in Roman Germany and excavation of those at Vetera (Xanten) and Novaesium (Neuss) has made a major contribution to the understanding of medical care in the Roman army. One room at Neuss contained more than 100 medical artefacts, which led to the conclusion that the large, rectangular buildings with corridors at legionary fortresses were hospitals[12,19]. A Roman cremation grave at Bingen contained a set of more than 60 bronze surgical instruments that, undoubtedly, belonged to a physician[10,11]. A Greek inscription to Asclepius, found at Cologne, is further proof of the presence of Greek-trained physicians (Asclepiads) in the Roman army[20]. There were many forts along the eastern border of Roman Germany and it is possible that further studies of these will also yield evidence of Aesculapius, *medici* and Asclepiads. Jackson records a collegium of doctors at Aventicum (Avenches, Switzerland), its presence referred to on a stone inscription set up by two of its members who were both *medici*. The name of one, Postumius Hermes, appears on an oculist stamp found 50 km away[21]. No dedication to Aesculapius has been recorded from this site but Aesculapius was worshipped at Augst in Switzerland[22].

Table 5a Archaeological evidence of 45 additional sites of Asclepian worship in Roman Gaul, Germany, Switzerland and Belgium

Location	No sites	Latin name
Twenty-nine sites recorded by Esperandieu[16]		
Aix-en-Provence	2478 & 80	Aquae Sextiae
L' Aire du Chapitre	2479	
Andelot	7188	
Arles	6705	Arelate Sextanorum
Avignon	451	Avenio
Basle	5488	Basilia
Bordeaux	1083	
Carmes	2645	
Darmstadt (Germany)		
Entains	2241	Intaranum
Hambach (Germany)	5127	
Laneuveville devant		
Nancy	4695	
Langres	3242, 3307	Andematunnum
Le temple du Monte de Sene	2170	
Lezoux		
Martres-Tolosanes	912 & 892	
Melam	2984	
Mesnie-sous-Lillebonne	308	Juliobona
Moulezan	6806	
?Narbonne		Narbo Martius
Nîmes	2648	Nemausus
Saintes		Mediolanum Santonum
Sainte Colombe	2605	
Sainte Fontaine pres de Merlebach	4442 & 4454	
Seurre	3587	
Vaison-la-Romaine		Vasio Vocontiorum
Vienne	2594 & 2602	Vienna
Vichy	2753	Aquae Calidae
Nine sites recorded by E Sikora[18] (and one possible site)		
Aoste		
Evaux-les-Bains		
Grenoble		Cularo
Godesberg (Germany)		
Mayence (Germany)		Moguntiacum
Obernburg (Germany)		
Orléans		
Cenabum		
Reims ?Asc	8389	Durocortorum
Trier (Belgium)		Augusta Trevorum
Seven additional archaeological sites from other sources[10,20-2] (and one possible site)		
Augst (Switzerland)		
Neuss (Germany)		Novaesium
Xanten (Germany)		Colonia Ulpia Trajana
Bingen (Germany)		Bingium
Cologne (Germany)		Colonia Claudia Ara Agrippinensium
Avenches (Switzerland)		Aventicum
?St-Rémy-de-Provence (France) (Spring to Valetudo)		Glanum

The *Edelstein Testimonies* include 21 additional sites located by epigraphy, none of which appeared in the review by Walton (Table 5b). Even the Edelsteins excluded some Latin inscriptions, especially those that were repetitive or of local interest only. There is a clear need to assemble all the relevant epigraphical material relating to Asclepius since the major publications, including *Corpus Inscriptionum Graecarum* and *Corpus Inscriptionum Latinarum consilio et auctoritate academiae litterarum regiae*, do not provide comprehensive coverage of all known inscriptions. The search should seek additional inscriptions to Asclepius, Aesculapius, Hygieia, Salus, Telesphorus, as well as those recording *medici* and *medicae*[23].

Table 5b *Edelstein Testimonies'* 21 additional sites from epigraphy

Location	Site	Location	Site
GREECE		ISLES	Thasus, Euboea
PHOCIS	Delphi	CRETE	Lebena
BOEOTIA	Erythrae	LYDIA	Between Mount Coryphe and a sea, Smyrna
ATTICA	Aegina, Cydantidae	CARIA	Tralles
ARGOLID	Philius	SYRIA	Beroea
ARCADIA	Halieis	LACONIA	Between Amyclae and Therapne, Megalopolis
PELOPONNESUS	Philius, Titane	SICILY	Acragas
ACHAIA	40 stades from Dyme and 80 stades from Patrae	ITALY	Croton, Antium

In Roman times, Hispania included present-day Spain and Portugal. Recent work has identified six additional dedications from this province (Table 5c). An inscription from Braga (Bracera Augusta) reads 'Asclepio et Hygiae', which used Latin script with Greek thinking as did one from Lisbon (Olisipo), 'Asclepio'; this format is similar to the one at Tunstall (Figure 64) and offers further evidence of Greek-trained Asclepiads serving in the Roman army[20,24–6].

Table 5c Six additional archaeological sites of worship in Roman Spain[24–6]

• Ampuria (Emporium)	• Santander
• Barcelona (Barcino)	• Cuidad Leon (Legio VII Gemina)
• Malaga (Malaca)	• Umeri (Salus Umeritana — Pyrenes)

The Athens National Museum contains two of the most famous bas-reliefs of the god of medicine; neither were listed by Walton. One is from Thyrea in Argolis (Figure 15) and the other from Oropos in Attica (Figure 66). The latter bas-relief (c400–350 BC) is unique as the inscription records that the patient, Archinos, gave the dedication to Amphiaraus at Oropos, who was a healing deity identical to Asclepius in appearance and methods. This diety gained favour during the Great Peloponnesian War (431–404 BC) and acted as a substitute for Asclepius.

A review of the bas-reliefs, votives and coins in the museums of Greece and other centres of the ancient world would, undoubtedly, identify additions to the Asclepian sites listed in Tables 5d and 5e.

Table 5d Twelve archaeological sites from miscellaneous sources

Location	Site
ALBANIA	Butrino (Buthrotum)[27,28]
BULGARIA	Glava-Panega (also coins)[29], Novae[13,14], Pernik[30]
CROATIA	Split (Diocletian's Palace)[30]
ITALY	Baiae (probable)[31], Ponte di Nona (probable)[32], Ostia[33], Fregellae[34]
AFRICA PROCONSULARIS (TUNISIA)	Bulla Regia[35,36], Thurburbo Maius[35,36], Jebel Oust[35,36]

Table 5e Twelve sites (uncollated material) from museums, collections and books

Source	Site
National Archaeological Museum, Athens	Argolis, Thyrea
	Attica, Oropos
Coin collections	Coins of Mabbott Collection: Adana in Cilicia[*37]
	CNG Catalogue: Moesia Inferior-Nikopolis ad Istrium[*38]
	Private collector: Pisidia-Codrula[*]
	Schouten: Acarnania, Astaeus[*39]
	Amorgos, Aigiale[*33,34]
	Storer: Cilicia, Anazarbos[*40]
	Wroth: Italy, Verona[*41]
	Thrace, Imbros[*41]
	Pautalia[*+42]
Books	*Pagans and christians*: Lydia, Oenoanda

*Coins as sole source of identification. Readers are invited to enlarge this list especially possible additions from Morocco and Algeria

+ Site identified in the BMC. Alice Walton lists Thrace, Pantalia, as a sole coin source. Map references show Pantalia to be in Sicily and no such place exists in Thrace. It is probable that her reference was a spelling error rather than a geographical error

Asclepian temple sites identified by coins

Coins of the ancient Greek world frequently identified their source of origin by depicting the predominant local deity. This practice has served to identify many Asclepian temple sites and sometimes the coin is the only remaining record of a temple's existence.

The Greeks depicted the head of Asclepius in frontal or profile views and portrayed him with full beard, mature features and a fillet in his hair. When standing, he is shown wearing a *himation* and is accompanied by his serpent-entwined staff. Seated views were less common, but always included an accompanying serpent and some-times a dog. Hygieia and Telesphorus could be substituted as identifying portraits for Asclepian temple sites and some later coins replaced one of his attributes, such as the serpent-entwined staff, a serpent-entwined omphalos, a cupping vessel or, occasionally, a symbol representing the master of the gymnasium. The portrait of the predominant local deity on coins may reveal the date the god became prominent in the geographical area of issue. It is surprising that Asclepius did not replace Heracles on the coins of Cos until 166 BC, 200 years after the death of Hippocrates.

In Roman times, the depiction of Salus on the reverse of coins was often accompanied by the inscriptions '*Sal*', '*Salus Aug*' or '*Publica*', which express a desire for the health of the state or emperor. This was an expanded sphere of influence for the daughter of Aesculapius and, when appearing on general issue coinage, did not identify sites of worship. Where Asclepius was not the predominant deity, the coinage would not indicate his presence. His portrait might also be used in 'alliance currency' which depicted the predominant deities of two city states to symbolize the economical or military alliance of the two regions (eg Asclepius of Pergamum paired with the Ephesian Artemis). Emperors occasionally assigned coins depicting gods from one area to another more for economical than religious reasons — these infrequent transfers can result in misidentification of temple sites. Despite these variables, the depiction of Asclepius on a coin from an identified locality in the Greek world usually identifies the site of an Asclepian temple as well as an archaeological artefact.

Romans continued this Greek tradition until 262 AD, when Emperor Gallienus (253–68 AD) reformed the imperial minting policy. He closed local mints in the eastern part of the empire, with resultant loss of coins with local religious flavour. This monetary reform limited coinage to standard designs minted under central control at designated centres. The new coinage continued to depict Asclepius and Salus, especially when the emperor had special need of their help. The most interesting example of this practice is a coin series of the usurper Carausius, who established the first 'British Empire' in 287 AD. His political and military situation was unstable and he needed to muster military and divine support. He used the inscription '*Salus Aug*' but, in addition to the traditional portrait of Salus feeding a serpent, made unique use of Aesculapius in this role by portraying him standing with his serpent-entwined staff. These coins, struck at both the London and Colchester mints[43], suggest considerable familiarity with Aesculapius in Roman Britain.

Coins and the 'index of cult sites'
Alice Walton reviewed the *Catalogues of Greek coins in the British Museum* and *Description de medailles antiques I–IV, Paris* 1807–37 by TE Mionnet[1]. Coins were associated with 220 of the 368 Asclepieia she identified (Table 2); for 164 of these, coins were the sole source of identification (Table 3). In 1966, Hart reviewed afresh the *Catalogues of Greek coins in the British Museum* and identified 161 Asclepian temple sites, 36 of which were not on Walton's list (Table 6)[44]. The identification totals by both Walton and Hart are underestimates of Asclepieia numbers as the London and Paris collections have accessioned additional specimens since the 19th century catalogues were published. Tables 5d and 5e include 10 additional sites identified by coins. There are probably other specimens of Asclepian coins not included in these tables; it is hoped that readers will provide additional data from other collections and catalogues.

Table 6 Thirty-six additional sites located from coins in the British Museum Catalogues

---

THESSALY to AETOLIA: Dyrrhachium
PONTUS, PAPHLAGONIA, BITHYNIA, KINGDOM OF BOSPHORUS: Amisus
TROAS, AEOLIS, LESBOS: Antandrus★
IONIA: Erythrae
LYDIA: Bagis, Germe, Stratonicea, Tripolis
CARIA AND DORIAN ISLANDS: Alabanda, Aphrodisias, Astypalaea, Heraclea
    Salbace
PHRYGIA: Alia, Amorium, Apameia, Sebaste, Trajanopolis
LYCIA, PAMPHYLIA, PISIDIA: Apollonia Mordeum, Conana, Etenna, Perga,
    Seleucia, Side, Termessus Major
LYCAONIA, ISAURIA, CILICIA: Elaeussa Sebaste, Epiphanea, Mopsus,
    Pompeiopolis
PHOENICIA: Berytus, Carne, Sidon
PALESTINE: Aelia, Neapolis, Tiberias
ITALY: Metapontum
ARABIA, MESOPOTANIA AND PERSIA: Esbus

★Lesbos: Walton listed Pordoselene but did not describe coins from there

This updated review locates a total of 513 sites associated with Asclepius (Aesculapius) (Table 7). Of the 267 Asclepian temple sites associated with numismatic material, coins provided the only source of identification for 211 (Table 8). The numismatic clues given in Tables 3, 5e and 6 are seeds for future archaeological discovery because coin evidence substantiates the presence of an Asclepieion more accurately than a simple dedication or an altar. This review of the locations of Asclepian worship demonstrates the practical value of numismatics to archaeology and emphasizes another research potential of coin collecting.

Table 7 Total number of Asclepian sites identified from all sources (coins, epigraphy and archaeology)

Walton (Table 2)	368
Additional sites from Britain (Table 4)	13
Additional sites from other sources (Table 5)	96
Additional sites from coins (BMC) (Table 6)	36
Total	**513**

Table 8   Summary of coin identification of temple sites

Coins associated with sites in Walton Review (Table 2)	220
208 different sites + 12 multiple sites	
Additional sites from BMC	37
(Table 6: 36 + 1)	
Other Sources (Tables 5d & 5e)	10
	Total 267
Coins as sole source of probable* temple location	
Walton (Table 3)	165
BMC (Table 6)	36
Other (Tables 5d & 5e)	10
	Total 211

* In Imperial times, coins were struck on behalf of the emperor and designs may have been transferred from one town to another

Impact of Aesculapius on politicians and philosophers

Coins demonstrate the political impact of Aesculapius. He had the approval of almost every Roman emperor and caesar who, between the years 54 and 324 AD, depicted the god of medicine on the reverse of at least one of their coin series (Table 9).

Some emperors minted the coins at time of ill health; this was especially true of Caracalla (211–7 AD), whose numerous temple visits suggest psychoneurosis rather than physical ill health. Others may have

Table 9 Roman emperors, empresses and caesars who depicted Asclepius or Salus on their coins (all dates relate to length of reign)

Nero	54–68 AD	Elagabalus	218–22 AD
Galba	68–9	Alexander Severus	222–35
Vespasian	69–79	J Mamaea	222–35
Titus	79–81	Maximinus	235–8
Domitian	81–96	Pubienus	238
Trajan	98–117	Gordian III	238–44
Hadrian	117–38	Philip I	244–9
Sabina	117–38	Trajan Decius	249–51
Aelius Caesar	136–8	Hostilian	251
Antoninus Pius	138–61	Valerian	253–60
Faustina II	146–75	Postumus	259–68
Marcus Aurelius	161–80	Gallienus	260–8
Lucius Verus	161–9	Victorinus	268–70
Lucilla	161–83	Aurelian	270–5
Commodus	180–92	Tacitus	275–6
Albinus Caesar	193–7	Probus	276–82
Septimus Severus	193–211	Carus	282–3
J Domna	193–217	Carinus	283–5
Geta	211–2	Diocletian	284–305
Caracalla	211–7	Carausius	286–93
Plautilla	211	Allectus	293–6
Macrinus	217–8	Maximianus	286–305
Diadumenian	217–8	Licinius	307–24

portrayed Aesculapius at the time of an epidemic. The coins depicting Salus on behalf of the general welfare of the Roman state or the emperor have already been described. All coins portraying Aesculapius were distributed beyond the Roman empire and were present wherever there was commerce. Many continued to circulate for centuries after the decline of the Roman empire.

Most academic giants of antiquity proclaimed their esteem for Asclepius and the words of these philosophers, historians, rhetoricians, poets, politicians and physicians are cited in the *Edelstein Testimonies*. Some are of particular interest. For instance, Plato recorded the dying words of Socrates: 'Crito, we owe a cock to Asclepius. Pay it and do not neglect to do so'. (Plato, *Phaedo* ET 524)

Sophocles accepted Asclepius into his house and set up an altar for him. After his death, the Athenians called Sophocles: 'Dexion [the one who receives] because of his reception of Asclepius; for he received the god into his house and set up an altar to him'. *Etymologicum Magnum* (ET 591)

The Neo-Platonists believed that Asclepius was the soul of the world, by which creation was held together and filled with symmetry and balanced union (ET 304). Pausanias recorded in *Descriptio Graeciae* (VIII, 28, 1, ET 549) that Alexander the Great dedicated his spear and breastplate to Asclepius at Gortys in Arcadia[45,46]; he also recorded that the sword of Memnon (the Ethiopian prince slain by Achilles at Troy) rested in the Nicomedian temple of Asclepius (ET 800). In 23 AD, Tacitus recorded that Tiberius confirmed the right of asylum to Cos (ET 798).

Aristides (129–89 AD), the Greek rhetorician and sophist, wrote on his own illness and on miraculous cures: '... the one who is guider and ruler of all things, the saviour of the universe and the guardian of immortals...'. *Oratio* XLII (ET 303)

Aristides explained his appeal to poets and writers with: '... give me as much health as I need for my body to obey that which my soul wishes...'. *Oratio* XXXVIII, 24 (ET 323) 'Here the stern cable of salvation for all is anchored in Asclepius'. *Oratio* XXIII, 18 (ET 402)

From Julianus (332–63 AD), we have: 'Asclepius heals our bodies, the Muses train our souls with the help of Asclepius and Apollo and Hermes...'. *Contra Galilaeos*, 235 B (ET 324)

In 53 AD, Emperor Claudius granted Coans immunity from taxes and declared their island a place sanctified only to Asclepius (ET 799). After the earthquake at Epidaurus in the first half of the second century AD, Senator Antoninus rebuilt the sanctuary and adorned it with magnificent monuments (ET 739). Soranus (second century AD) wrote: 'Hippocrates, by birth, was a Coan... who traced his ancestry back to Heracles [Hercules] and Asclepius, the 20th in descent from the former, the 19th from the latter'. *Vita Hippocratis, 1* (ET 216)

Galen (129–99 AD) recorded the contemporary building of the temple of Zeus Asclepius at Pergamum (ET 803). He also wrote: '... the ancestral god Asclepius, whose servant I declare myself to be, for he saved me when I was suffering from a deadly condition of an abscess'. (ET 458)

Epigrammata Graeca 1027 (second to third century AD) (ET 598) exhorted: 'Wake, Paeon Asclepius, lord of men...'.

Asclepius was everywhere in literature and everyone was familiar with his deeds. In the second century AD, he stood at the peak of his power and influence and was known throughout the ancient world. He became identified as Imhotep Asclepius in Egypt, Eshmun Asclepius in Phoenicia, Zeus Asclepius at Pergamum and Jupiter Aesculapius in Rome[47,48]. One might have justifiably hailed him as Aesculapius Optimus Maximus.

Many of his temples occupied highly prestigious locations, such as the Acropolis at Athens and at the city of Carthage as well as the island in the Tiber at Rome. Through their association with the Roman army, the Asclepiads introduced Aesculapius Castrorum to the far northern and western limits of the Roman world. His influence was ubiquitous and indeed Aesculapius was everywhere from Memphis in the south to Carpow in the north; from Ecbatana in the east to Wales in the west (Map 2).

Map 2   Geographical distribution of Asclepian sites from all sources

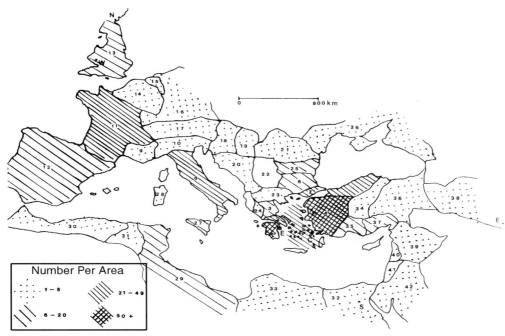

drawn by Buhle

Numbers indicate ancient name and brackets indicate modern region

1. Peloponnesus (southern Greece; E = location of Epidaurus)
2. Attica
3. Thessaly (eastern peninsula of central Greece)
4. Asia (western part of Asia Minor which included Mysia, Lydia, Caria, Phrygia, Troas & Ionia); P = the site of Pergamum
5. Aegean Islands and Doric Islands; C = island of Cos
6. Thracia (central & south Bulgaria)
7. Pontus (north-east Turkey)
8. Italia (Italy)
9. G Narbonensis (Provence region of France)
10. G Cisalpina (north Italy)
11. Gallia (France)
12. Hispania (Spain & Portugal)
13. Britannia (England, Wales, parts of Scotland)
14. Belgica (Belgium)
15. Germania Inferior (northern Germany)
16. Germania Superior (southern Germany)
17. Alpes & Noricum (Switzerland, Austria & parts of neighbours)
18. Pannonia Superior (western parts of Hungary & former Yugoslavia)
19. Pannonia Inferior (eastern parts of Hungary & former Yugoslavia)
20. Dalmatia (Adriatic coast of former Yugoslavia)
21. Dacia (Romania)
22. Moesia Superior (Serbia)
23. Macedonia (northern Greece)
24. Epirus (north-west Greece)

25. Moesia Inferior (north Bulgaria)
26. North of Black Sea (southern Ukraine & east Georgia)
27. Sicilia (Sicily)
28. Sardinia (Sardinia)
29. Africa (province which included Algeria, Libya, Cyrenaica, Mauretania & Egypt)
30. Mauretania (Morocco & part of Algeria)
31. Numidia (Algeria)
32. Aegyptus (Egypt)
33. Cyrenaica (eastern Libya)
34. Galatia (central Turkey)
35. Lycia & Pamphylia (southern Turkey)
36. Cappadocia (eastern Turkey)
37. Cilicia (southern Turkey)
38. Media (western Iran)
39. Syria (Syria)
40. Phoenicia (Lebanon)
41. Judea (Israel)
42. Arabia (north-western Arabia)

W = Brecon, the westernmost evidence for Asclepius
N = Carpow, the northernmost evidence for Asclepius
S = Memphis, the southernmost evidence for Asclepius
E = Ecbatana, the easternmost evidence for Asclepius

Notes and references

1. Walton A. *The cult of Asklepios*. New York: Ginn & Co for Cornell University Press, 1894. Reprinted by Johnson Reprint Corporation, New York and Johnson Reprint Co Ltd, London, 1965. Sources of material (literary, epigraphic, archaeological and numismatic) are fully referenced in this work.

2. This inscription was probably removed from the Roman fort that was located two miles away at Overborough (Galacum) and placed in the western jamb of a window in the nave of the Parish Church of Saint John the Baptist at Tunstall, Lancashire.

3. Collingwood Bruce JB. *The Roman wall*. 3rd edn. London: Longmans, Green, Reader and Dyer, 1867: 264.

4. Collingwood Bruce JB. *The Roman wall*. 3rd edn. London: Longmans, Green, Reader and Dyer, 1867: 238.

5. Jackson R. A Roman healer god from Sussex. Report of the acquisition by the British Museum of a statuette from Chichester depicting Asclepius. *J Brit Mus Society* winter 1995; **23**: 19–21.

6. *The Roman baths and museum*. Bath: Bath Archaeological Trust, 1990.

7. Scarth HM. *Aquae solis, notices of Roman Bath*. London: Simpkin Marshall & Co, 1864.

8. Page W, ed. *Victoria county history for Kent: no 3*. London: St Catherine's Press, 1932: 116.

9. RCHM (England). An inventory of historical monuments in London. *Roman London* 1928; **3**: 151.

10. Wiseman J. A visit to ancient Glanum. *Archaeology* 1998; **51**(6): 12–8.

11. Elbe JV. *Roman Germany: a guide to sites and museums*. Mainz: Verlag Philipp von Zabern, 1977: 61–5.

12. Jackson R. *Doctors and diseases in the Roman empire*. London: British Museum Press, 1988: 134–5.

13. Koléndo J. Le culte des divinitiés Guérisseuses à novae. *Archeologia* (Polish Academy) 1982; **33**: 65–78.

14. Bosilova V, Koléndo J, Lesznk M. Inscriptions latines de novae. *Éditions scientific de l'Université Adama Mickiewicz de Poznán*, 1992.

15. Field NH. *Dorset and the second legion*. Tiverton: Dorset Books, 1992.

16. Esperandieu E. *Recueil general des bas-reliefs, statues et bustes de la Gaule Romaine*. Republished in 1966 by Gregg Press Ltd, Hants, England. The 15 volumes include: Tome premier (T1), Alpes Maritime, Paris, 1907; T2, Aquitaine; T3, Lyonnaise, Premier Partie, Paris, 1916; T4, Lyonnaise, deuxieme Partie, Paris, 1913; T5, Paris, 1915; T6, Belgique, Deuxieme Partie, Paris, 1915; T7, Gaule Germanique, 1 Superieure, Paris, 1918; T8, Paris, 1922; Tome neuvieme, Gaule Germanique, Inferieure, Paris, 1925; T10, Paris, 1922; T11, Supplement and general inclusive index, 1938; T12, 1947; T14, supplement V, Belgie V; T15, 1966. *Recueil générale des bas-reliefs, statues et bustes de la Germanie Romaine*, Paris and Brussels, 1931.

17. Esperandieu E. *Epigraphie Romaine*. Libraire des Ecoles Françaises d'Athens et de Roma du Collège de France & de l'Ecole Normal Supérieux du Poitou & de la Saintonge, 1889, Ernest Thorn, Paris; Saintes, 1888; des Limovices, 1891; de Lectoure, 1892; Narbonnaise, 1929, Ernest Laroux, Paris.

18. Sikora E. Le Culte D'Esculape en Gaule. *RAC* 1983; **22**: 175–84.

19. Pitts LF, St Joseph JK. *Inchtuthill*. London: Britannia Monographs, 1985.

20. Galsterer B, Galsterer H. Die Romischen Steinschriften aus Köln, *Wissenschaftliche Katalogue des Romisch-Germanischen Museums Köln*. Köln: Greven & Bechtold, 1975.

21. Jackson R. *Doctors and diseases in the Roman empire*. London: British Museum Press, 1988: 85.

22. Jackson R. *Doctors and diseases in the Roman empire*. London: British Museum Press, 1988: 160–3.

23. Some of the epigraphic references used by Walton: *Corpus Inscriptionum Latinarum consilio et auctoritate academiae litterarum regiae*. Berlin: Borussicae editum, 1863; Boeckh A. *Corpus Inscriptionum Graecarum*. Berlin, Borussicae editum, 1825–77; *Corpus Inscriptionum Atticarum consilio et auctoritate academiae regiae litterarum*. Berlin: Borussicae editum, 1873; Dittenberger W. *Corpus Inscriptionum Graecarum Graecae Septentrionalis*. Volume 1. Berlin, Borussicae editum, 1892.

24. Vivres J. *Inscriptiones Latinas de la Espagna Romana*. Barcelona: Universidad de Barcelona, departmentos de Figogia Latina, 1971.

25. Santos FD. *Inscripciones Romanas de la Provincia de Leon*. Imprime Grapicas Celarayn SA. Poligona Industrial de Leon.

26. Fabre G, Mayer M. *Epigraphie Hispanique*. Paris: Publication du Center Pierre Paris, Diffusion E., De Boccard, 1984.

27. Ugolini L. Butrino. *Antiquity* 1935; **9**: 104.

28. *The London Times* January 1 1935: 13.

29. Kazarow G. The Thracian rider and St George. *Antiquity* 1938; **11**: 295.

30. Kraljevic C. The temple of Aesculapius in Diocletian's palace at Split. *Lijenicki Vjesnik* 1995; **117**(3–4): 7–102.

31. Jackson R. *Doctors and diseases in the Roman empire*. London: British Museum Press, 1988: 56.

32. Jackson R. *Doctors and diseases in the Roman empire*. London: British Museum Press, 1988: 160–1.

33. Calza G, Becatti G. *Ostia*. 4th edn. Rome: Instituto Polygraphico Dello Stato, MCMLVIII.

34. Crawford MH, Keppie L (with contributions by Mattingly DJ, Mudd P). The sanctuary. *Proc Brit Sch Rome* 1984; **52**: 24–32.

35. Hinton A, ed. *Blue guide Tunisia*. 1st edn. New York: WW Norton, 1996: 111–3, 212–5.

36. Personal communication: Mrs Merry Ross.

37. Holzer H, ed. The Hans MF gallery. *Coins of the Roman world*. New York: Thomas Ollive Mabbott Collection, Parts I and II 1969.

38. Lancaster PA. *Classical coins*. CNG March 30 1994: 925.

39. Schouten J. *The rod and serpent of Asklepios*. New York: Elsevier Publishing Company, 1967: 47.

40. Storer HR. *Medicina in numis*. Boston: Wright and Potter Printing Co, 1931.

41. Wroth WW. Telesphoros. *J Hellenic Studies* 1882, **3**: 283–300.

42. Penn RG. *Medicine on ancient Greek and Roman coins*. BA Seaby and Classic Numismatic Publications, 1994.

43. The mint mark 'C' on Romano-British coins has been interpreted as Colchester (Camulodunum). There has been some debate about its representing Southampton (Clausentum) by Gilbert Askew in: Askew G. *The coinage of Roman Britain*. London: BA Seaby Ltd, 1951. Conversely, Richard Reece suggests that the Roman 'C' sometimes looks like a G and the mint represented could be Glevum (Gloucester): Reece R. *Coinage in Roman Britain*. London: BA Seaby Ltd, 1987.

44. Hart GD. Ancient coins and medicine. *Can Med Assoc J* 1966; **94**: 77–89.

45. Alexander's dedication of his spear and breastplate to Asclepius was in thanks for Asclepius saving his life. He received a near fatal chest wound at the battle against

the Malli, when an arrow penetrated his corselet and entered his body above the breast. The blood from the wound was mixed with air breathed out from the pierced lung. Alexander collapsed with shock; some authors state that the arrow was cut out by Critodemus, a doctor from the island of Cos and of the family of Asclepius. This is an excellent description of a penetrating chest injury and the doctor was an Asclepiad who knew how to treat this potentially fatal condition[44].

46. Arrian. *Life of Alexander the Great.* Translated by Aubrey De Selincourt. Middlesex: Penguin Books Ltd, 1962.

47. Bartlow RM. The origin of the caduceus. *Aesculapius* 1971: vol 1, no 1. Bartlow has suggested that Eshmun of the Phoenicians may have had a link with early Egyptian medical healing rituals. The Egyptian god, Ptah, cured disease in the third millennium BC by sleep visitation and dream therapy. Ptah became god of prophesy and healing and was adopted by the Phoenicians and other peoples in the eastern Mediterranean. In the seventh century BC, Imhotep the physician was deified and became the son of Ptah. The early Egyptian gods, Uzoit, Nikhbet and Thoth were depicted with a single serpent entwining a staff. Were Eshmun-Asclepius and Imhotep-Asclepius a coincidence or a divine circle? Did early Greek traders take the Egyptian concept of healing back to Greece or did the Asclepius cult develop *de novo* in Greece?

48. Asclepius had numerous other epithets. 'Soter' or saviour was popular and was even inscribed on some of the coins of Pergamum. People's level of regard for him was shown by their use of the epithets 'Philanthropotatos' (the most manloving), 'Euergetes' (benefactor) and 'Philolaos' (friend of the people). His religious status was shown in Zeus-Asclepius, Dominus, Deus, Augustus and Paeon (who was the original physician to the gods). His medical role is recalled in 'Cotyleus' (of the hip joint) at Therae with reference to curing Hercules of a wound inflicted by the Hippocoon and his sons. The 'Castrorum' was a reference to the army doctors (Asclepiads) revering him and using his services to assist with wounds, illnesses and injuries. Alice Walton listed, with references, 55 additional Greek epithets. Perhaps one of these epithets was used to describe his additional role as the veterinary god.

Chapter 10

Asclepius and Christianity

Asclepius was worshipped by every echelon of society in the Graeco-Roman world. His ever-expanding prestige and influence reached its zenith by the middle of the third century AD but, after this date, his popularity began a gradual and progressive decline. Meanwhile, Christianity began to emerge as the predominant religious force. This change may well have been facilitated by the existence of the many striking similarities between Asclepius and Jesus Christ.

Christ and Asclepius: some theological parallels

Both Christ and Asclepius had a heavenly father: Christ was conceived by the Holy Ghost and Asclepius was the son of Apollo. On the other hand, each had a mortal mother. The birth of each reflected its heavenly origins. Christ was conceived by the Holy Ghost and carried in the womb of a virgin. Asclepius was conceived in the womb of the fair maid Coronis and was delivered from his dead mother's womb by Apollo, who performed a caesarian delivery as her funeral pyre had been lit. Furthermore, the births of each were associated with divine light: that of Christ was heralded by the appearance before shepherds of heavenly angels with the glory of the Lord shining around them and also by a brilliant star in the east. According to Pausanias who wrote in the second century AD, a shepherd discovered the infant Asclepius and he saw a divine light all around the child (ET 7).

The mothers of both Christ and Asclepius, following conception, were associated with mortal males: Mary was 'adopted' by Joseph, despite his being 'minded to put her away privily'; Coronis, possibly in an attempt to legitimize her pregnancy, took Ischys, the son of Elatus, or the 'youth of Thessaly' as her lover (ET 1 & 2). According to Homer, Asclepius had been a living physician who became a hero-god and, at a later stage, a full god related to the Olympians. Christ also began his life on earth. Asclepius and Christ led blameless lives dedicated to the succour of humanity. They did not fight wars or perform heroic deeds. They were said to have taught love and compassion and the authors of antiquity recorded their ability to heal both body and soul alike: '... Asclepius both restores the souls of sinner and the bodies of the sick'. Julianus (332–63 AD) *Contra Galilaeos*, 200 A-B (ET 307)

Worshippers of Asclepius and Christ were rewarded with health and salvation; Asclepius linked treatment to purity of the mind while Christ linked treatment to eternal salvation. Both were able to perform miracles that cured disease: 'When we say that he [Jesus] made well the lame and those with paralysis and those who had suffered poor health from birth and that he raised people from the dead, we shall be referring to deeds that are just like and even identical with those said to have been performed by Asclepius'. Justinus (second century AD), *Apologia*, 22, 6 (ET 94)

Christ and Asclepius were both prosecuted under the law of the day and died a mortal death. Their death sentences were carried out to satisfy the demands and jealousy of dissatisfied members of their own religious establishments. Christ had disobeyed the basic Jewish law that prohibited work on the Sabbath day when he healed a cripple at the Pool of Bethesda with the miraculous words: 'Rise, take up thy bed and walk' *St John* (New Testament of Holy Bible; chapter 5 verse 16). These words and actions raised the ire of the Hebrew clergy who had to persistently argue with Herod to convince him that Christ had behaved unlawfully: 'The Jews persecuted him and sought to slay him because he had done these things on the Sabbath day' *St John* (New Testament of Holy Bible; chapter 5 verse 8). Christ died on the cross and his death was accompanied by a lightning storm in the heavens. Asclepius was punished following a complaint from Hades, the god of the underworld, to Zeus that his realm was becoming depopulated due to Asclepius reviving the dead. Zeus executed the successful physician by hurling a thunderbolt from heaven and he was subsequently turned into a constellation of the northern hemisphere (Ophiuchus).

After their deaths, Christ and Asclepius were resurrected. Christ returned to the earth as part of a heavenly plan and as a sign to his followers; Asclepius was resuscitated to continue the medical care of mankind with the proviso that he would desist from raising the dead. Both were gods who lived among mankind—Christ was a divine human and Asclepius a terrestrial divinity.

Both possessed 'divine hands': Asclepius' were his drugs and light touch in healing, while Christ's healed by touch or blessed and consecrated men for his service. They also had strong family associations: Christ with his mother, Mary, and Asclepius with his daughter, Hygieia.

Christ and Asclepius were each part of a Holy Trinity. Christ was associated with the Father, the Son and the Holy Ghost. Asclepius was third in descent from Zeus, being the son of Apollo who, in turn, was Zeus' son. He was '. . . the one who is guide and ruler of all things, the saviour of the universe and the guardian of immortals and ... overseer of the helm of government, he who preserves things which are eternal and those that are about to come to pass'. Aristides (129–89 AD), *Oratio* XLII, 4 (ET 303)

Both Christ and Asclepius were considered saviours and associated with the salvation of man. Today, use of the term 'saviour' to describe any other than Christ may be considered by some to be blasphemous. This opinion has resulted from centuries of Christian religious insistence on the uniqueness of Jesus Christ, but the term is not the exclusive domain of Christ and was applied to Asclepius in the second century BC. This appellation was even proclaimed on some of the coins from Pergamum which bore the inscription '*Soter*' (Greek for Saviour) (Figure 12a). A saviour provides salvation and Aristides wrote in the second century AD: 'Asclepius is the sheet anchor of salvation for all humanity'. Aristides (129–89 AD) *Oratio* XXIII, 15–8 (ET 402) (For an alternative translation see chapter 9.)

Christians linked the treatment of disease to salvation because they felt sickness of the body was a reflection of sickness of the soul. It is interesting also to note that 'purity of the mind' was required of all supplicants to Asclepius before they could be healed. Both required faith from their followers. The Greeks abhorred reasoning based on faith but their belief in the Greek pantheon needed faith and success of much of the Asclepian temple medicine required faith. Even today, a gram of faith in a doctor may be worth a kilogram of pills.

During the first three centuries of our era, Christ was depicted as a young man without a beard. His earliest known appearance in mosaic was found at the fourth century AD Roman villa of Hinton St Mary, Dorset, England. Here, his face is identified by an accompanying chi rho symbol and a pair of pomegranates signifying eternal life (Figure 69). The modern concept of the face of Christ is similar to the ancient depiction of Asclepius which portrayed a mature man with a full head of hair, a beard and a kindly demeanour. Papadakis wrote in 1988 that, during the fourth century AD, a statue believed to represent Christ was found at the foot of Mount Hermon in the town of Paneas (Caesarea Philippi)[1]. Alice Walton lists this as the site of an Asclepian temple on the basis of coinage issued under the country division of Samaria. The Panean 'Christ statue' depicted a mature man with kindly face, beard and a full head of hair. This sculpture was probably a depiction of Asclepius from the Asclepieion of Paneas and may have inspired the face of Christ that predominated in art after the middle of the fifth century AD. The incorrect identification of this statue could explain the artistic change from the youthful Christ depicted in Figure 69 to

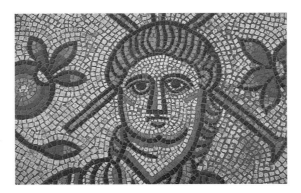

Figure 69 Earliest mosaic portrait of Christ depicting a youthful face with the chi rho symbol and pomegranates. This was excavated at Hinton St Mary, Dorset, England, dated to the fourth century AD. (The mosaic is in the British Museum. Photo courtesy Roger Peers, the Dorset County Museum, Dorset, England)

the familiar bearded face that many generations of worshippers have associated with him.

It should be no surprise that this long list of similar attributes shared by Christ and Asclepius constituted a sharp challenge to the rigid orthodoxy of third century church leaders. If it were not for the existence of contemporary documentation, even today's reader might find these statements hard to accept. When the Christians began their battle against the pagan gods for the souls of humankind, 'Asclepius was the leading deity in the struggle between the dying world of the pagans and the rising world of the Christians' *(Edelstein Testimonies II Interpretation*, page 111).

Christianity: from persecution to prominence

Christianity began as a small religious sect in the first century AD. Its appeal, despite adversity, progressively increased until it was adopted in the fourth century as the official religion of the Roman empire. This growth occurred regardless of Christian refusal to obey the laws of Rome, which required all citizens to propitiate the gods who preserved and protected Rome. The followers of Christ were rigid in their belief in one god and refused to recognize the deities of Rome. When challenged by the authorities, who required this worship, they showed their defiance, preferring to face martyrdom. Artists even refused to create images of the old gods or to decorate their temples. Records exist of Diocletian's visit, in 293 AD, to the province of Pannonia (roughly coterminous with modern Hungary). He had ordered the construction of new Asclepian temples and the execution of Christian

stone masons working in a porphyry quarry because they had refused
to make a statue of Asclepius and Diocletian[2,3].

By the third century, the Roman empire had weakened from years of
internal power struggles. Capable leaders had been killed, national
wealth had been squandered and disruption of industry, trade and
capital investment existed[4]. Emperor Diocletian (284–305 AD) tried
addressing these issues by instituting a series of reforms that included
return to the divine and absolute power status of the emperor. He
proclaimed his own descent from Jupiter and citizens were required to
worship him and prostrate themselves in adoration before an audience.
The Christian refusal to do this initiated the most widespread
persecution of the Roman era[5]. Their churches were razed and their
sacred books burnt; their property was confiscated and they were
pursued by infuriated mobs. They were imprisoned, enslaved and
tortured, and many Christians were martyred. Almost by divine
serendipity, the antiChristian policy failed and their brave acceptance
of a horrible death became a source of inspiration to many. This
resulted in growing numbers of new converts who believed that they
would inherit the kingdom of God after death.

The very conditions that Diocletian failed to correct provided fertile
ground for proselytization by the Christians. Jesus offered hope and
eternal salvation for all. Many of the early converts were among the
uneducated classes that knew the hardships of daily life well. Their very
existence relied on faith in the fruitfulness of the annual harvest or in
'something turning up' to sustain their lives. For those who lived in
rural areas and whose lives were so precarious, the words of *Matthew*
had particular appeal: 'It is easier for a camel to pass through the eye of
a needle than for the rich man to enter the kingdom of God' (*St
Matthew*; chapter 19 verse 24); 'But many that are first shall be last and
the last shall be first.' (*St Matthew*; chapter 19 verse 30).

Christ tolerated all sinners and absolved their sins. Such a concept
would have been abhorrent to the elite in society, who believed that
those entering the temples of Asclepius had to be pure in thought and
deed. Their views were shaken by the aftershock waves of the
earthquake that destroyed the Asclepian sanctuary at Pergamum
c252–60 AD. Christians viewed the disaster as fulfilment of the
prophesy given in the message of Saint John the Divine to the angel of
the church in Pergamum which stated:

'And to the Angel of the Church in Pergamon write: these things
saith he which hath the sharp sword with two edges. I know thy
works, and where thou dwellest, even where Satan is: and thou

holdest fast my name and hast not denied my faith, even in those days wherein Antipas was my faithful martyr, who was slain among you where Satan dwelleth.' (*Revelations* II, 12, 13)

'Repent or else I will come unto thee quickly and will fight against them with the sword of my mouth.' (*Revelations* 16, 11)

Sinners who did not repent at other churches named in the book of revelation were also threatened with violent and malicious punishment. Christians preached that the destruction of Pergamum was an example of the power of God. The impact of temple destruction was more than physical as, regardless of the prestige of the Asclepieion of Pergamum, no attempts were made at reconstruction. Instead, the most important Asclepian sanctuary in Asia suffered the ultimate indignity of becoming a burial ground. In the same decade as the earthquake, traditional followers of Asclepius experienced another blow to their confidence by the scandal surrounding association of Asclepius with the charlatan Alexander of Abonoteichus (referred to in chapter 3). It fell to Constantine 'the Great', who was proclaimed 'Caesar' in 306 AD, to continue to search for ways in which the empire might be bolstered. Following his early military consolidation, he courted the support of the growing body of Christians by recognizing their faith and, thus, paving the way for establishing Christianity as the official religion of the later Roman empire.

Constantine the Great

Constantius, Augustus (emperor) of the western Roman empire, died at York in 306 AD. The British legions proclaimed his son as their new emperor but Galerius, emperor in the eastern half of the empire, reluctantly agreed to bestow on Constantine the subordinate title of 'Caesar'. This decision averted immediate civil war and allowed him time to consolidate his political and military position[6]. Constantine was a talented strategist who believed he had a divine purpose to become sole ruler of the Roman empire. His religiosity brought about two religious visions that influenced his political career. The first of these occurred in 309 AD at the temple of Apollo Granno, the healing deity of the Gauls[7]. While Constantine was asleep in the sanctuary, Apollo and the goddess Victory appeared and promised him 30 years of success and happiness. As a result, Constantine believed he enjoyed a close association with Apollo and proclaimed this to the people by minting special coins depicting Apollo, with the inscribed message '*Soli Invicto Comiti*' (to the unconquered sun [Mithras/Apollo] my friend) (Figure 70). These coins were first minted in 310 AD and continued to

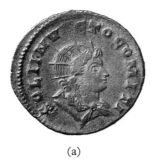
(a)

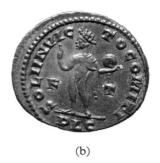
(b)

Figure 70   Coins of Constantine inscribed 'SOLI INVICTO COMITI' dedicated to the 'unconquered sun (Mithras or Apollo) my friend'. (a) Radiate and draped bust of Sol (Apollo) struck 310–3 AD at Trier mint. (b) Sol standing holding a globe in his left hand struck at Lyons mint after Constantine had adopted Christianity (c312–9 AD) (GDH)

be made until 318 AD, six years after Constantine's acceptance of Christianity. They were used throughout the empire long after Constantine's death.

His second vision occurred in 312 AD immediately before his critical battle at Milvian Bridge, the outcome of which would decide political supremacy in the western empire. This time, Constantine saw in the noon sky a 'sign of the cross' inscribed with the words 'by this, conquer'[8] (Figure 71). That night, he dreamt that Christ commanded him to use its likeness in his engagements with the enemy. The

following morning Constantine adopted a new battle standard comprising a cross surmounted by a combination of the first two Greek letters for 'Christ', XP (chi rho). This combination of letters is described today as 'the Cross of Constantine' and the entire standard (*labarum*) is still used as a symbol of Christ (Figures 72 & 73)[9].

He also placed a cross on the shields of his soldiers who fought and conquered Maxentius under the Christian banner; by virtue of his victory, Constantine became the uncontested Augustus of the western Roman empire. After his success, he erected a large statue

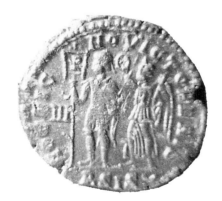

Figure 71   Coin minted at Siscia in 350 AD by Vetranio signifying his allegiance to Constantius II. The reverse depicts Constantine holding a labarum and being greeted by Victory. It is inscribed 'HOC SIGNO VICTOR ERIS' (by this sign thou shalt conquer) (GDH)

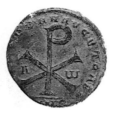

Figure 72 Reverse of a coin minted by Magnentius at Amiens in 351–2 AD which depicts the Christogram (chi rho) symbol for Christ (the first two letters in the Greek word for Christ). This is flanked by the Greek letters alpha and omega, which were Christian symbols for beginning and end respectively. The inscription around the rim reads 'Salus DD NN Aug et Caes' which translates as: 'The health of Caesar and Augustus, our lords'. This is an un-Christian attitude towards the heads of state but, by this time, the chi rho symbol had also become a symbol of imperial government and the accompanying α and ω had replaced the depiction of Salus as a symbol of the health to the emperor and state (GDH)

of himself holding the cross, or 'sign of salvation', in the Roman basilica of his defeated rival Maxentius. He also funded the erection of the church of St John the Lateran and his mother, Helena, founded the Sessorian basilica. The sign of the cross was now visible on the skyline of Rome. His first significant political gesture towards Christians occurred with the Edict of Milan that was signed in 314 AD by himself, as emperor of the west, and by Licinius who, by now, had become the emperor of the east. This charter gave official recognition to Christianity throughout the Roman empire.

Licinius' support of the edict was one of convenience and he resumed persecution of eastern Christians in 321 AD; in the west, however, Constantine continued to encourage Christians and gained their political support by granting tax immunities and making other enactments favourable to them. He also corrected the injustices of his predecessors and restored the property that Christians had lost through persecution. Cooperation between the two emperors deteriorated and, in 324 AD, another civil war began to fulfil their personal ambitions of establishing one supreme Augustus of the Roman empire. Licinius was defeated and eventually sentenced to death. Constantine demonstrated his absolute power and religious policy by minting many coins that portrayed a Christogram on their reverse, rather than representation or symbols of a pagan god. He adopted benign contempt for paganism; it was no longer the official religion of the state and worship of the old gods was regarded as a mere superstition.

To facilitate the Christianization of the Roman world, Constantine planned an impressive new capital at Byzantium. Many cities, including some of those mentioned in the New Testament, had

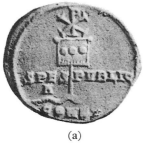
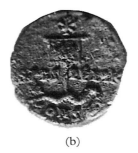

(a)   (b)

Figure 73
(a) Bronze coin of Constantine minted at Constantinople (326–30 AD), depicting a *labarum* impaling a serpent. The *labarum*, the standard adopted by Constantine after his conversion to Christianity, consists of a purple silk banner hanging from a crosspiece on a pike. A chi rho symbol of Christ surmounts the staff. The inscription '*Spes Publica*' translates as 'Hope of the Populace' and the symbolism refers to the replacement of Asclepius by Christ. The front half of the serpent shows an interesting pattern of localized wear which may be the result of rubbing it as a talisman against disease; this wear pattern parallels that demonstrated on the serpent of the Chichester figurine (Figure 23). Alternatively, the wear may reflect the effect of repeated derogatory gestures made towards the serpent as a symbol of evil (Photo HKC, M&W; reproduced courtesy of Spink and Sons, London, England)
(b) A specimen of this rare coin was found at Wroxeter. Its importance would be greatly increased if excavations of the recently discovered, extensive archaeological remains disclose evidence of an Asclepian temple (Photo Dr Roger White and Mr Richard Brickstock)

competed for this honour. His final choice was based on political and strategical reasons, but he was able to make this palatable to the various religious and civic authorities by claiming that the location was a divine choice that had been revealed to him in a dream. Construction of Constantinople began in 324 AD and the city was dedicated to the Blessed Virgin on 11 May 330 AD. After this date, Rome, with its many pagan monuments and history of debauchery and intrigue, epitomized the past and Constantinople symbolized a new era for the Roman empire. This was proclaimed on a coin minted at Constantinople that inscribed '*Spes Publica*' (Hope for the People). It also showed a *labarum* impaling a large serpent (Figure 73a), a depiction which meant more than the triumph of good over evil as serpents, symbolic of Asclepius, had been portrayed on currency of the Mediterranean lands for the previous 700 years. This coin proclaimed the end of the prominence and power of Asclepius, and the adoption of Christianity and a new era for the empire[10].

As Constantine's Christian beliefs matured, he used his position of power and authority to indulge his love of oratory. He preached at length, to both theological and political audiences, that his own successes and his enemy's failures were living examples of the divine will of God. He wrote letters or epistles to the provinces of the empire, which emphasized the surety of divine punishment for those who had persecuted the church and of rewards for those who pleased God. His words spread the gospel of Christianity and bonded Christians to him. Robin Lane Fox summarizes this with the words, 'The moral crusader from Britain claimed to have swept the world with the guidance of God'[8].

Constantine's conversion to Christianity emanated from his devout belief in a supreme deity, but his vision of the 'sign of the cross' did not result in the development of a zealous evangelical fanatic. Quite to the contrary, his subsequent behaviour even suggested some ambiguity in his commitment. For instance, he continued to mint the '*Soli invicto*' coins for six years following his conversion to Christianity. His triumphal arch, constructed in Rome and dedicated in 315 or 316 AD, did not demonstrate any recognition of Christ[11]. This was probably a shrewd omission to avoid offending Rome's military and political establishment who were staunch followers of paganism. At the inauguration of Constantinople in 330 AD, a statue of Apollo—its head replaced by that of Constantine—was hoisted to the top of a column in the forum. This action suggests that Constantine still revered Apollo's appearance to him in the vision of 309 AD and believed that he still retained a personal association with the god.

Constantine preached religious tolerance toward pagans and believed that Christians must learn to live with them as neighbours. His tolerance of paganism during his climb to the top may have been pure pragmatism to retain the support of the establishment who still believed in the old gods. Perhaps he did not understand the true depth of Christian religious dogma that gained strength as a result of his support and became an overtly intolerant and maliciously destructive force against paganism.

Constantine continued to be involved in wars and to eliminate political opposition. Taken ill in 337 AD, he was treated at the baths at Helenopolis and died in Nicomedia[12]. Perhaps Asclepius had the last word—if the former Asclepian temple of Nicomedia had still been functioning, he might have recovered!

Was it serendipity that Constantine died in the 29th year after Apollo had promised him 30 years of success and happiness? Very significantly, he was not baptized until the time of his death. The baptism may have been delayed so he might die free of sin, but his unbaptized condition raises serious doubts about the depth of his Christian convictions. During his many campaigns, he was at risk of the sudden death that would have denied him entry into heaven.

Perhaps his consummate skill at political manoeuvring was the reason for his postponement of baptism. This procrastination over his ultimate acceptance of Christianity on a personal basis would have encouraged church leaders to continue to cooperate with him; at the same time, he could remind them of the temporal side of his favour and their religious freedom. This policy would also have encouraged the pagan factions of the empire to give him continued support to enjoy religious tolerance and to avoid persecution for their beliefs.

The epithet 'Great' was bestowed on Constantine due to his political successes in reorganizing the Roman empire and his foresight in gaining the support of Christianity. In addition, he made himself and his family 'Great' by creating the dynamic absolutism of his family — the 'Gens Flavia'. Constantine understood the potential political force of Christianity and exploited it to secure his goals[13]. He also understood the virtues of religious tolerance and, in that respect, he was a great man many centuries ahead of his time.

Subtle persuasion also contributed significantly to the success of Christianity as many churches were built on the sites of pagan temples and pagan practices were adapted and modified to appear Christian[8]. Pagan festivals were important in the ancient world as they represented the only official breaks in the daily work routine. Many were also adopted into the Christian calendar and the choice of Sunday (Sol's day) as an official weekly day of rest would, itself, have been a favourable attraction to pagans and Christians alike. The polytheistic tradition of associating individual deities with particular attributes was maintained in the adoption of various saints with specialized powers and their particular gifts were often acquired as a manifestation of their martyrdom. Wealthy patrons of the church gave lavishly for the construction of buildings which used the power of architecture to attract followers; they sponsored pilgrimages, supported holy men and made donations for ornate church furnishings. All this was carried out with the desire of focusing attention on the church and of assuring their own eternal life.

The Christians also converted 'pagan' festival days into Christian holidays; in fact, even the supposed birth date of Christ replaced the Mithraic feast in honour of the same 'Sol invictus' who appeared on the coins of Constantine (Figure 70)! Did Constantine influence the church when it adopted the feast day of Sol invictus as the birthday of Christ?

Decline of Asclepius

Paul, in his first epistle to the Corinthians, emphasized the unity of all parts of the body and likened this unity to the body of Christ. He illustrated his words by examples of the foot, ear, eye, hand, head and the uncomely parts; these examples were carefully chosen and may well have alluded to the votive body parts displayed in the Asclepieion of Corinth (I *Corinthians* 12: 12–31). His words initiated doubts about the sanctity of votives in Asclepian temples. Despite this, the popularity and worship of Asclepius continued until the middle of the third century AD. At this time, the hitherto impregnable loyalty of his followers was weakened by the exposure of his reputed grandson 'Alexander of Abonoteichus' as a charlatan and by the earthquake that destroyed Pergamum, thus fulfilling a Christian prophesy. Perhaps 'the sword coming out of the mouth' in chapter 2 of *Revelation* was a metaphor for the pen being mightier than the sword (ET 330). Church leaders began an unremitting attack on Asclepius, as part of a general attack on all things pagan, and words from many of their tirades have survived: '. . . he had been instructed by the priests of Asclepius, the god who does not heal souls but ruins them'. Eusebius Hieronymus (c348–420 AD) *De Vita Hilarionis*, 2 (ET 330)

'Here is someone who has been aroused by the stirrings of an evil spirit; he rages, he is mad: let us take him into the temple of... Asclepius or Apollo. May the priest of either, in the name of his god, bid the evil spirit to come out of the man: no way can that happen.' Lactantius (fourth century AD) *Divinae Institutiones*, IV, 27, 12 (ET 333)

Asclepius' scholarly supporters rallied to his defence: 'And when he [the devil] presents Asclepius as one who raises people from the dead and who heals other diseases, may I not say that in this respect also he has imitated the prophesies that were made about Christ?' Justinus (second century AD) *Dialogues*, 69, 3 (ET 95)

'. . . they are amazed that disease has afflicted the city for so many years, now that Asclepius and the other gods no longer dwell there. For it is a fact that since Christ has been held in honour, none of the gods have enjoyed a single bit of support.' Theodoretus (393–457) *Graecarum Affectionum Curatio*, XII, 96–97 (ET 506)

Constantine gave his subjects physical evidence of his support to the Christians when, at a bishop's request, he sanctioned the destruction of the Asclepian temple at Aegae. The war of words became a war of destruction; once Christianity became an accepted religion, its leaders changed from benign representatives of a gentle Christ to intolerant and scheming persecutors. The destruction of the temple at Aegae is well recorded and typical of such events in the fourth century.

The new attitude towards the old gods and especially towards Asclepius is revealed in the writings of Eusebius of Caesarea (Eusebius Pamphili c260–340 AD). He was the most erudite historian of his time and is best known for his *History of the Christian church*, which contains an explanation (*apologia*) for the history of Christianity with proof of its divine origin and efficacy. In his writings, he embellished Constantine's dream of the cross into a miraculous apparition that appeared as a flaming cross in the midday sky proclaiming 'by this conquer'. He also singled out Asclepius as the major enemy of Christianity and wrote in *De Vita Constantini*, III, 56 (ET 818):

'In regard to the god of the Cilicians, the deception of men who were seemingly wise was very great, with thousands getting all worked up about him as if he were a saviour and a physician who sometimes revealed himself to those who were asleep [in the temple]. At other times, he healed sickness of those whose bodies were sick but he was thoroughly destructive of souls, drawing people away from their true saviour and leading astray into godless ways those who were of a dishonest inclination. The emperor [Constantine], therefore, acting justly and believing the true Saviour to be a jealous god, gave orders that this temple, also be razed to its foundations. One nod of the head and the building lay demolished on the ground. That famous place that had been the wonder of the noble philosophers was overthrown by the hand of a soldier — and with it fell he who lurked there, not a spirit nor a god, but a kind of beguiler of souls, who had practised his deceit for many a long year. Then, the very one who offered his services to rid others of evils and misfortunes could find no remedy with which to protect himself. For the story goes that he was struck with a thunderbolt. But not in the realms of mythology was the just action of the Roman emperor who found favour with God. It was clear for all to see that the righteousness of the Saviour himself had brought about the complete destruction of the temple in that place in such a way that not a single trace of those former crazy goings on was left.'

The stones and columns from the temple were used to build the Christian church at Aegae. The fifth century church historian, Sozomenus, also stated in *Historia Ecclesiastica* (ET 819) that: 'at that time [in 331 AD], the temple of Asclepius at Aegae was raised to the ground and vanished completely'. The fate of the temple at Aegae was symbolic of the fate of many Asclepian temples and the rumble of its destruction was the death knell of Asclepius. A dedication made in 355 AD to Asclepius at Aegae was found at Epidaurus; this might have been an 'In Memoriam' or a prayer for its re-establishment by Julian who had just been made Caesar.

During his brief reign, Emperor Julian, the Apostate, attempted a return to paganism[14]. He became Caesar in 355 AD but did not become sole Augustus until November 361. He died in battle against the Persians after only 18 months in power and did not have time to complete his reforms. His failure (or near success) was typified by the records of Zonaras in *Epitome Historiarum* XIII, 12C-D (ET 820). Julian had ordered the high priest of the Christian church built at Aegae to return the pillars that had been taken from the Asclepian temple. With great difficulty, one pillar was taken down and transported to the doorway of the church but could not be moved further. The work was eventually abandoned and, when Julian died, the bishop restored it to its place in the church. The bishop seemed to know that the return to paganism would fail—he only made a token effort to remove the columns. He probably used the death of Julian as another example of the righteousness of Christianity.

This was the last formal attempt to halt the growth of Christianity and restore the status quo of old gods. What would have happened if Julian had lived long enough to implement his reforms? For how long would the old gods have survived?

The continuing decline of paganism and Asclepius was gradual[15]. Many Asclepieia became Christian centres. The temple on the island in Rome became the forerunner of the present-day church of San Bartolomeo del Isola and a church for the Healing Saints was built over the sanctuary at Athens. Also, a church dedicated to the healing Saints Cosmas and Damian was built over the temple at Corinth and a shrine to St Therapon replaced the Asclepieion at Mytilene; a small part of the basilica at Epidaurus was converted into the church of St John. Some Asclepian temples survived into the sixth century, notably the one at Cos which remained active until its destruction by an earthquake in 554 AD.

The neoplatonist Proclus, who died in 485 AD and who supported Asclepius, had some remarkably modern thoughts about doctors: 'But it is to mortals that the medical art which derives from theory and experience must be assigned; by this means some people master the divine art of healing to a greater extent, others to a lesser degree' (ET 312). A continuing Hippocratic school at Cos may have influenced his thoughts which remain true today—some doctors are better than others. Proclus' biographer, writing in the fifth century, reveals that the Asclepieion at Athens was still functioning even though the sanctuary of Athena at the Parthenon had become a Christian church:

'And Proclus . . . went up to the Asclepieion to pray to the god for the ailing girl. For it is a fact that the city [of Athens] at that date still rejoiced in the presence of this god and still had the temple of the Saviour intact . . .' Marinus fifth century AD, *Vita Procli*, chapter 29 (ET 582)

The fifth century writer, Theodoretus, suggested continuing clandestine worship of Asclepius: 'You honour him with both libations and sacrifices, once you did this in the open but now you do it in some secret corner'. (ET 5) But no-one knows when the last prayer was offered to Asclepius, and there are some today who still believe that he can cure.

Notes and references

1. Papadakis T. *Epidauros*. 7th edn. Zurich: Verlag Schnell & Steiner, 1988: 9.
2. Diocletian set about reforming and revitalizing the empire. He was able to stop the self-destruction resulting from power struggles between legions and provincial governors. He stabilized the administration by establishing a tetrarchy with an augustus (emperor) in the east and another in the west; each had a successor and heir who governed with him under the title Caesar. He reformed the currency and attempted to establish price control. However, he failed to recognize the benefits that might accrue from gaining the support of growing numbers of Christian believers. On the contrary, the Christians were perceived as disloyal to the Roman gods and, as such, constituted a threat to the wellbeing of the empire.
3. Mocsy A. *The provinces of the Roman empire: Pannonia and Upper Moesia*. Translated by Sheppard Frere. London: Routledge and Kegan Paul, 1974.
4. Coin hoards reflect times of insecurity. The discovery of large numbers of buried coins serves as a window on the past. It is possible to date their time of burial from the mix of coins present; many such hoards dating to the third and fourth centuries AD have been discovered throughout the Roman empire.
5. It was not until the mid-third century that Roman authorities instituted a systematic and vigorous persecution of Christians. Earlier outbursts, such as Nero's infamous attack following the fire of Rome in 64 AD and the throwing of Christians to wild beasts in the amphitheatre at Lyons in 177 AD, may be regarded as responses to particular circumstances. By the third century, however, increasing concerns about the stability of the empire highlighted the need to deal with disloyalty and intransigence of Christian believers.
6. At this time in Roman history, a separate augustus (emperor) and a subordinate caesar ruled the eastern and western divisions of the empire.
7. 'The most beautiful temple in the world' was the temple of Apollo Grannus at Grand in eastern Gaul: King A. *Roman Gaul and Germany*. London: British Museum Publications, 1990: 143. This temple possessed baths and an amphitheatre and practised incubation. Although the Gauls did not adopt Asclepius, their 'Apollo' had many of the attributes of Asclepius.
8. Lane Fox R. *Pagans and Christians*. London: Penguin Books, 1988. This encyclopaedic work by an award-winning Oxford historian should be read by all

those interested in this period of transition in world history. Lane Fox notes that it was not an exceptional event and that modern sunwatchers have often reported the sighting of cross-shaped haloes. It is to be hoped that this statement has not encouraged his readers to test this observation by directly gazing at the sun without the protection of welder's glasses. Direct viewing of the sun for even half a second may burn the most sensitive part of the retina, resulting in permanent or temporary damage. It is likely that the 'cross-shaped haloes' seen are the result of retinal injury.

9. The chi rho sign was not used in a Christian context before Constantine's vision[8], but this device (an abbreviation for the Greek 'chreston') was used on pagan papyri as a method of drawing attention to the contents of a paragraph. This was the ancient counterpart for underlining, marker, NB or boldface type. Perhaps Constantine purposely invented this new use for a familiar pagan symbol with a double meaning of 'Take note, Christ'.

10. One of these coins was found at Wroxeter, England (Figure 73b). (Richard Brickstock: personal communication.)

11. The arch of Constantine is one of the best-preserved monuments of ancient Rome; Christian symbols are still absent.

12. Constantine. *Encyclopaedia Britannica* 1946; **6**: 297–300.

13. This section is only intended to be a summary of Constantine's life and influence, and is a personal interpretation of his actions.

14. Julian was given the epithet 'Apostate' meaning one who has renounced his religious faith. He had been educated by Eusebius, Bishop of Nicomedia, and was trained as a Christian. He became attracted to the old faiths and especially to the idea of joining paganism with philosophy.

15. Some Christian churches that replaced Asclepian temples, like the one at Aegae, were probably built more as a display of triumph than for pure spirituality. They maintained the continuity of holiness and worship at the island in the Tiber, and preserved the staff of Asclepius and his portrait (chapter 7). The temples of other pagan cults popular with the Romans — such as Mithras, Isis and Serapis — were also attacked and destroyed. Malicious, purposeful destruction has been demonstrated at the temples of Mithras at Carrawburgh on Hadrian's Wall and at Wallbrook in London. The use of ancient buildings as stone quarries for subsequent structures has resulted in many churches of today containing interesting remnants of the past. The example of the nave at the parish church of Saint John the Baptist in Tunstall, Lancashire, England, has been mentioned in chapter 9; the external walls of Whitchurch Canonicorum contain Roman tiles, discussed in chapter 11. The practice of erecting churches over the destroyed remains of pagan temples has left a potential storehouse of architectural features that may be revealed when church buildings require under-pinning, the installation of central heating or other structural changes[16,17]. Geomagnetic surveys using magnetometers, radar enhancement and computers were used by Casey, Noel and Wright at Lanchester (Longovicium) to reveal the subsoil topography of the Roman fort[18]. It is possible that these techniques could be adapted to reveal details of buried structures without damaging overlying buildings. These techniques will be most useful in modern British towns built on the sites of Roman ones. Christians built their churches (which often became cathedrals) on the sites of Roman temples; such temples, usually located at the site of the main cross roads of a Roman fort, then became the centre of both the Roman town and the subsequent British one[19].

16. In the winter of 1966–7, a grave weakness was discovered in the foundations of the central tower of York Minster. The task of architectural reinforcement was

combined with archaeological investigation. As a result, the central hall of the *Principia* building (headquarters) of the Sixth Legion was discovered and has been preserved in the newly created undercroft. (Cant R. *The undercroft York Minster*. London: Pitkin Pictorials Ltd.) This could have been the room where Constantine was proclaimed Augustus in 306 AD.

17. In the winter of 1993, the central heating system at Canterbury cathedral was being replaced; simultaneous archaeological studies revealed that the earlier Saxon cathedral was much larger than previously conceived. The full report is not yet published.

18. Casey PJ, Noel M, Wright J. The Roman fort at Lanchester, County Durham: a geophysical survey and discussion of the Garrisons. *Archaeol J* 1992; **149**: 69–81. It is of interest that the survey did not reveal a structure that could be interpreted as the hospital. This was the site of a dedication to Asclepius which was inscribed in both Latin and Greek (chapter 7).

19. Wacher JS. *The towns of Roman Britain*. London: BT Batsford Ltd, 1974.

Chapter 11

Asclepian heritage

This chapter describes the influence of Asclepius on Christian traditions and chapter 12 reviews the modern legacy of ancient medical practice. The remarkable spread of Christianity was aided by the subtle adoption of many pagan religious customs; foremost among these are the contributions of Asclepius, the healer and saviour. The full influence of pagan religions on Christianity has been described in Robin Lane Fox's encyclopaedic work *Pagans and Christians*[1].

Continuity of sanctity

Many sacred areas of the world have an aura of mystery and holiness. These places are usually located on summits, in dells and forest clearings, beside streams, pools, springs, caves and amid ancient ruins. Over the ages, a diversity of gods has been worshipped in such places and the offering of prayers has created an almost tangible atmosphere of spirituality and reverence. Worshippers of Asclepius practised continuity of sanctity when they built their earliest temples on obsolete shrines to Apollo; subsequent sites were endowed with natural beauty as well as an ample source of natural spring water. Christians used the aura of many pagan holy sites to attract converts and continued to apply the healing powers of sacred springs which they re-named after their own local saints. They destroyed the shrines of pagan deities and reused the rubble as their source of building materials; hence, fragments of Roman masonry are to be seen frequently in the walls of ancient churches[2,3]. Many Roman building structures, for example the Jewry Wall in Leicester, have remained due to their being incorporated into Christian buildings. Although building materials could, in many cases, have been obtained from ruins of a neighbouring Roman building, it is possible that many will have derived from an original pagan shrine that had been destroyed or abandoned.

The church of San Bartolomeo, on the island in the Tiber at Rome, is an outstanding monument to the continuity of sanctity between Asclepius and Christianity. The temple of Asclepius on the Insula was described in chapter 7; there is, however, a hiatus in the records between the fall of Asclepius and the ninth century, when Benedictine monks established a hospice here for pilgrims travelling to Rome. At the end of the 10th century, Emperor Otto III built on the site a basilican-style church dedicated to Saint (St) Adelbeit (Albert) that contained the relics of St Bartholomew and St Paulinus. Columned arcades of rich black marble, probably originating from the Asclepian temple, divide the nave. The brothers of the Order of St John of God replaced the Benedictine monks on the island in 1584. Their Order became known as the Fatebenefratelli (translated as 'do well brothers') and they continued to care for the sick at a hospital that became known as the Ospedale (Hospital) Fatebenefratelli. The present church of San Bartolomeo is the result of restoration carried out in 1624[4].

Belief in the healing powers of St Bartholomew's relics was so great that, in the 11th century, the church was re-named after him. The sacred spring of Asclepius became the healing spring of St Bartholomew and its original location the centre of the nave, at the foot of the chancel steps leading to the altar. In the 13th century, a new marble parapet was installed over the opening to the well; this depicts on its sides the bas-relief figures of Christ, St Albert, St Bartholomew and Otto III (Figure 74). The marble brim of this wellhead has smooth, deep grooves caused by centuries of friction from stout ropes drawing up the curative waters for distribution to Christian supplicants.

The Ospedale Fatebenefratelli is located on the upper segment of the island and currently possesses 420 beds housed in a 17th century building. It features a cool, central colonnaded courtyard where patients and staff enjoy the air and soothing ripple of water trickling from a fountain into a shallow pool. Below ground level, there is a new, state-of-the-art diagnostic imaging department. The corridor leading to the magnetic resonance imaging equipment provides a spectacular example of ancient and modern construction living cheek by jowl. Archaeologists supervised the construction of part of the basement so that any ancient remains discovered could be preserved and displayed. Parts of the new corridor floor are made from tempered plate glass through which the walls of the original Asclepian temple complex can be seen. No lift is present at the western end of this corridor as construction would have required demolition of ancient stone walls; instead, staff, patients and the odd privileged visitor descend a stairway bounded by temple walls. The hospital recently converted a 100-bed ward of the 18th century into a sophisticated, ornate lecture theatre used for international meetings and symposia. Today, the hospital is Rome's favourite obstetrical facility and more babies are born here than at any other city hospital; it is also listed in the *AA essential explorer*[5] as having one of Rome's best emergency departments. The hospital also serves as the motherhouse of the Hospitaller Order of St

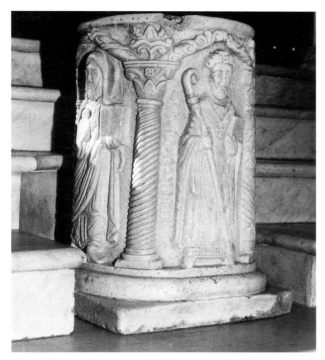

Figure 74 The new marble parapet (13th century AD) over the sacred well of St Bartholomew. The original sacred spring of Asclepius became the sacred well of St Bartholomew. Note the grooves caused by wear from ropes around the rim (Photo kindly supplied by the late Fr Flavian Keane and taken by the Photographic Department of the Ospedale Fatebenefratelli, Rome, Italy)

John of God that maintains international connections and sponsors medical aid to developing countries.

The Asclepian historian, Kerenyi, asked: 'What impelled the Romans to select this island, which could never have been healthful, for a temple and hospital dedicated to Aesculapius?'[6]. The answer to this question is continuity of sanctity. The island has a palpable atmosphere — the lingering aura of a tradition of religious patient care that has continued without interruption for 23 centuries.

A marble depiction of the staff of Asclepius from 292 BC, carved on part of the original boat-shaped temple of Asclepius, has survived the desecration of pagan symbols by early Christians. It symbolizes not only Asclepius but also continuity of healthcare and, as such, forms the logo of healthcare providers in Rome and around the world (Figure 53). The island was fertile soil for the seeds of religious tolerance advocated by Constantine and these have continued to germinate[7,8]. The Order of St John of God and its Ospedale Fatebenefratelli continues to 'do well' (*fate bene*) in Rome and around the world.

Rahere, an English monk, is the most remembered person to be cured by the sacred spring of Asclepius and St Bartholomew. Rahere was a jongleur when, following the death by drowning of Henry I's son in 1123 AD, he went on a pilgrimage to Rome[9]. While there, Rahere developed a fever (possibly malaria) and was treated at the Pilgrim's Hospice of St Bartholomew. Thinking that he would die, he vowed that, if he were allowed to go home, he would erect a hospital for the restoration of poor men and, as far as he could, would administer to the needs of the poor gathered there[10]. He prayed and drank the water of the sacred well. His recovery was rapid and, on his way home to London, he experienced a vision in which St Bartholomew appeared and directed him to build a hospital and church outside the city boundary at Smedfield ('flat field', present-day Smithfield). This was not an ideal location for a hospital as the land was marshy and it was the site for hanging criminals; despite this, funds were found and the hospital of St Bartholomew and the church of St Bartholomew the Great were opened in 1129 AD. Rahere had not been an educated man but became an Austin (Augustinian) Canon after his return to England; he was the first prior of the church, which came under royal protection. The 'book of foundation' of the church and hospital recorded instances of minor miracles and faith healing that occurred as a result of prayers said to St Bartholomew[10]. The hospital continues to serve the people who work and live in the city of London and has earned an international reputation for treating leukaemia and other diseases. St Bart's (as it is now often called) London has developed a special liaison with the Fatebenefratelli Hospital on Tiber island[11]. Recently, politicians and healthcare administrators tried to close the facility, but St Bart's continuity of sanctity and healthcare has been preserved by the unity of spirit of innumerable citizens, patients and professionals accompanied by a giant effigy of Rahere[12].

Songs, incense and purity

Asclepian religious services featured singing by the congregation, use of incense and the prerequisite of purity — Christianity adopted these rituals.

The historians MP Nillson and J Kroll believe that: '... the daily ceremonies of Asclepian temples deeply influenced the formation of the Christian service. The pagan reverence of old, which accentuated the sacrifice of animals, was gradually replaced by a more spiritual worship in which songs and bloodless offerings became increasingly popular'[13,14]. The regularity of divine singing addressed to Asclepius indicates that song was an integral part of his worship. If correct, then

Asclepian worship would form an important link between pagan and Christian ritual; from earliest times, hymns were an integral part of Christian ceremonial[15]. The chorus in the Greek play 'Plutus' sang: 'I shall sing with all my might to Asclepius, blest with his offspring, he who brings great light to mortals'. Aristophanes, *Plutus* lines, 639–40 (ET 277) These words resemble those of some songs of praise sung in today's churches. 'Anyone who enters the sweet-smelling temple must be pure; to be pure is to think only holy thoughts' was a guiding inscription at Epidaurus. Porphyrius, *De Abstinentia, II*, 19 (ET 318) 'The sweet-smelling temple' could also describe the churches of today that burn incense as an integral part of the ritual for Mass. 'Purity means to think nothing but holy thoughts' suggests a soul cleansed of sin and the quotation itself reminds of Christ's words quoted in one of the gospels: 'except ye come as little children ye shall not enter into the kingdom of heaven.' *Matthew*, 18, 3

Supplicants to Asclepius had to be physically and spiritually cleansed before seeking help. This was accomplished by bathing in the facilities provided at the temple; Christianity substituted an immersion ritual in the baptism ceremony. A detailed analysis of the origins of baptism is given in *Pagans and Christians*[1].

Right of sanctuary

Many Asclepian temples enjoyed the right of sanctuary that gave criminals protection from the law; however, Roman law did not grant this to Christian churches until the end of the fourth century. Many variations of the ritual continued until the 17th and 18th centuries. In 1623, King James I of England abolished the right of sanctuary but, due to legal loopholes, it lingered until 1723. Today, at Durham Cathedral, a replica of the sanctuary knocker is on the main door and tour guides delight in telling a variety of stories about the custom[16].

Christianity and coins

Greek coins depicted various gods to identify their place of origin and to authenticate their value, while Roman rulers portrayed various deities on coins to gain divine favour or to give a political message. These customs bestowed a religious purpose on coins that could also 'spread the gospel'. Constantine recognized this ancillary function of money when he minted coins honouring Apollo (Figure 70) and when he used coins from Constantinople both to consolidate the city as the new capital of the Roman world and to encourage conversion from old religions to Christianity. Coins with Christian icons neutralized the influence of circulating currency that proclaimed many of the ancient gods, especially Asclepius. The unique symbolism of Constantine's *'spes publica'* coin, minted before the formal dedication of Constantinople, was described in chapter 10 (Figure 73).

The coins of his successors continued to proclaim Christianity. One minted c350 AD by his son, Constantius II, depicts Constantine holding a *labarum* and is inscribed *'Hoc Signo Victor Eris'* ('by this sign thou shalt conquer') (Figure 71). Magnentius minted a 'salus' coin that depicted the chi rho symbol flanked by alpha and omega (Figure 72); between 346 and 361 AD, his successors celebrated the 'New Era' that became Byzantium, with the inscription 'Fel Temp Reparatio' (*felicium temporum reparatio* — 'happy times are here again'), echoes of FD Roosevelt's 'New Deal'[17].

Although the Byzantium empire began with the establishment of Constantinople as the new capital of the eastern Roman empire in 330 AD, it did not become a distinct cultural and political entity until the reign of Justin I (517–65 AD). Byzantium was a distinct, Greek-speaking, Christian nation based on Roman law and Roman civic organization[18]. It became the cultural and intellectual centre of the Mediterranean world and its great wealth assured the wide circulation of its coins that displayed Christian icons. The obverse of sides of Byzantine coins depict Christ, or the reigning monarch accompanied by various Christian symbols, and the reverse always carries a Christian message.

One of the best examples of this Byzantine tradition is a gold coin from Constantinople, minted during the reign of Basil II and Constantine VIII (976–1025 AD). On the obverse, it depicts Christ wearing a *nimbus cruciger, a pallium* and a *colobium* with his right hand raised in benediction while the left hand holds the *Book of Gospels*; the two monarchs are placed on the reverse, holding a cross between them[19]. Michael IV (1056–7) minted a gold coin showing Christ on the obverse with the inscription 'Jesus Christ, King of the Rulers'. The reverse depicts Michael at his coronation being crowned by the Virgin Mary, patron of Constantinople; this is an outstanding example of the artistic excellence of Byzantine numismatic art[20]. For more than 1,000 years, every Byzantine coin carried Christian symbols such as crosses, angels and saints, in addition to portraying Christ.

Christian symbols were also used on the coinage of other European nations, predominantly from countries belonging to the holy Roman empire. An outstanding example of this practice is illustrated by a coin minted by Emperor Thierry V von Boppert (1363–84), from Metz, which depicts a benediction by a bishop who is wearing his ceremonial regalia and his mitre on his head. His right hand is raised, the thumb and first two fingers extended, and his left hand holds his ceremonial crooked staff or crosier[21].

British coins depicted the cross from the eighth century until the introduction of decimal 'new pence', which began minting in 1968 but were dated for circulation in 1971[22]. Present-day portraits of Queen Elizabeth II continue to bear the inscriptions 'DG' (*Dei gratia*) and 'DF' (*Defensor fidei*) (by the grace of God and defender of the faith).

In medieval times, popes and bishops who acquired political power minted their own coins; these sometimes depicted their own portraits instead of Christ[23]. The progress of the crusaders was commemorated on coinage that celebrates their victories and even includes imitations of Arabic coins with pseudo-Kufic legends; however the cessation of these coins was a mute testimony to their defeat[24].

Salus, the daughter of Aesculapius, survived the fall of paganism. She is depicted on an early coin of the Christian era that was minted by Fausta, the second wife of Constantine I; this shows on the reverse a 'baptized' version of Salus, portrayed without a serpent but holding two children. The users of this coin would receive a cryptic message that the daughter of Aesculapius has repented and been converted to Christianity. Salus continued to be synonymous with the concept of health, wellbeing and political stability and appeared on coins that depicted the cross and were inscribed *Salus Mundi* (health and wellbeing of the world).

Christianity, more than any other religion, endowed coins with a religious role[25-7]. This practice served to spread and consolidate the influence of Christianity, in much the same fashion as the coins of Epidaurus and Pergamum contributed to the fame of Asclepius.

Christian religion and healing

As already discussed in previous chapters, the early Greeks and Romans understood illness as punishment from the gods but, in later times, their physicians believed that disease was caused by an imbalance of the body humours. Such imbalance was treated by physiological, conservative, symptomatic and religious therapy.

Christians believed that disease of the body reflected a sickness of the soul caused by sin or divine purpose, and that some illnesses were caused by demons that had to be expurgated by prayer and the use of charms. Christ was considered a physician and *Christus medicus* was the healer of sin. Their physicians combined prayers for the soul with treatment of the body; in the Middle Ages, they even believed that changing the body humours could affect the soul, so that it would develop love for God and for one's neighbour. Followers of both

Asclepius and Christ believed that healing could be accomplished by prayer, faith, touch and divine miracles.

Healing saints

A divine retinue (chapter 2) treated the ancient Greeks while Christians satiated an innate appetite for diversity in divine care by adopting various saints who performed miraculous cures of specific diseases. The saints accomplished cures by petitioning the supreme deity on behalf of the supplicant and by means of a therapeutic power that emanated from their tombs, or even from reliquaries containing their body parts, pieces of clothing or other associated artefacts. Their portraits and statues, like those of Asclepius and Hygieia, were also believed to possess specific curative powers. Sometimes, patients placed written petitions at the base of a statue of a saint, thus mimicking the practice of placing scrolls at the feet of Asclepius[28]. In some modern countries, help is still sought by sleeping at the base of a saint's statue, a remarkable re-enactment of the Asclepian incubation ritual. Shrines of the Virgin Mary and other healing saints are often decorated with crutches, orthopaedic appliances and other medical paraphernalia that have been left as votives of thanks by cured patients. These gifts, like the votives at the Asclepian temples, offer massive reassurance and hope to others seeking cure. Many Asclepian healing springs, as well as those of other pagan gods, were adopted by Christianity and re-named after a local saint.

First healing saints: Cosmas and Damian

Cosmas and Damian were twins born in an ancient area of modern day Turkey, who became physicians practising medicine and surgery during the later part of the third century AD. They were devout Christians treating their patients without fees in the hope that they would convert to Christianity. They travelled around the ancient world and were reputed to have practised on Tiber island that was sacred to the Roman gods Janus, Jupiter, Aesculapius and Vediovis. After the Emperor Diocletian (284–305 AD) reorganized the Roman empire and accorded to himself the status of a god who had to be worshipped, Christians, among them Cosmas and Damian, refused to obey. As a consequence, they suffered persecution from the authorities. Lycias, the Roman proconsul in Cilicia, ordered Cosmas and Damian to sacrifice to the gods of Rome; when they refused to do this, they were sentenced to death. The angels of the Lord protected them from death by stoning, burning and drowning; eventually in 287 AD, they were beheaded and buried at Cyrrhus in Syria, where their tombs became a place for cure and pilgrimage. Emperor Justinian I (518–27 AD) is reputed to have been cured of an illness at their tomb, which he commemorated by the dedication of the church of Saints Cosmas and Damian at Constantinople. This was built in the style of an Asclepian temple, and its operation also reflected Asclepian practices for the saints appeared to the sick while they dreamed. Five other churches were dedicated to them in Constantinople, which also practised nocturnal 'incubation'.

Pope Felix IV (526–30 AD) also honoured the twin physicians by building a church beside the forum of Rome. It was here that the two saints gained their greatest fame when they re-appeared in human form and performed miraculous surgery on the gangrenous leg of the sacristan of their church. They amputated the diseased limb and replaced it with a transplant leg from an Ethiopian who had died of old age and been buried in the church of St Peter ad Vincula. This miraculous surgery was a favourite subject for medieval artists — paintings by Fra Angelico (c1432) and Fernando del Rincon (16th century) hang today in the Museo di San Marco at Florence and Madrid's Prado respectively[29–32]. The surgical feat was as extra-ordinary as any of the miraculous surgeries described by those sleeping in the *abata* of Asclepius' temples. It matched, in extravagance, that of the woman with dropsy (fluid swelling of the body) who had her head cut off, was turned upside down so the fluid could be drained out and, after the tissues and body cavities were dry, had her head sewn back on (ET 423).

The sick continued to pray to Sts Cosmas and Damian in much the same way as supplicants appealed to Asclepius and Hygieia. The twins became the patron saints of physicians and pharmacologists in the fourth century AD, until the 16th century. In medieval times, they became the patron saints of the ancient Society of Barber Surgeons of London. After the reformation, the staff of Asclepius replaced the icons of Sts Cosmas and Damian. The Royal Society of Medicine continues to recognize them where they are supporters in their coat of arms. St Cosmas wears a blue physician's robe and holds in his right hand a pharmacy jar, while St Damian wears a red robe and holds a surgeon's knife with his left hand (Figure 75)[33]. This is discussed further in chapter 12.

Saints with a specialty
St Michael had been recognized as a general slayer of disease since the early days of Christianity. After the reformation, apothecaries reverted to using Apollo for this role, where he was placed in the centre of the

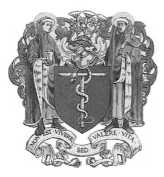

Figure 75 The coat of arms of the Royal Society of Medicine depicting Sts Cosmas and Damian supporting a tau cross entwined by the brazen serpent of Moses. The crest of the coat of arms depicts the medicinal herb betony (Reproduced with courtesy of the Royal Society of Medicine, London, England)

arms of the Society of Apothecaries and was depicted slaying the dragon of disease on the reverse of 17th century apothecary token coins[34].

Some saints acquired special powers with specific diseases. St Sebastian, for instance, became the patron saint of the bubonic plague through adaptation of the myth that credited Apollo's arrows with the ability to inflict and cure this affliction. Sebastian's martyrdom by arrows in the amphitheatre, therefore, bestowed on him the ability to relieve the plague. Subsequently, a church was dedicated to him on the former site of the temple of Apollo in Rome. Other protectors against the plague were St Roch (or Rock), who had recovered from the plague, St Anna, St Augustine of Hippo and St Fabian.

As St Anthony had special powers over the devastating symptoms of ergotism, the disease became known as St Anthony's Fire. St Lucia, St Odilia and others were patron saints of eye diseases. Many saints acquired their special healing roles from the method of their martyrdom. St Agatha, having had her breasts cut off, became the patron saint of breast feeding and breast diseases. She is depicted as bearing her severed breasts in a dish. St Apollonia became the patroness of toothache after her teeth had been knocked out by pointed stones; her emblem is a pair of forceps holding a tooth. Healing saints proliferated greatly during the Middle Ages and each became associated with a specific disease[35,36].

Many churches dedicated to Sts Cosmas and Damian practised 'incubation' with visitation, touching and cure during sleep. The ritual at churches dedicated to other saints involved sleeping near their bones or relics. Incubation was used in the early Christian church and continued into the Middle Ages, when 'incubation became a widespread cherished custom in Europe as well as Asia Minor and Egypt'[28]. This Asclepian custom was also used in Byzantium at the churches of St Cyrus, St John and St Therapon; the nearby church of St Michael at Sosthenium also cured by incubation. Churches known to have offered incubation facilities at Byzantium provided greater capacity for patients to undergo '*incubatio*' than any Asclepian centre of the ancient world! There were incubation facilities in Alexandria at the church of St Cyrus and St John, and some patients were cured by this means at the church of St Thecla at Seleucia in Isauria and by St Martin at Tours[28].

Medieval pharmacy

The ancient texts of Hippocrates, Galen, Dioscorides, Largus and others were preserved and copied by the monks. Their classical prescriptions continued to play an important role in the Christian treatment of the physical component of disease. Monks cultivated herb gardens at their monasteries, believing that the healing properties of their plants came from God's earth. These gardens, which have been portrayed in art and described in literature, were the medieval counterpart of the courtyard herb garden of the Roman *valetudinaria*. Visitors to the ancient town of Shrewsbury can see a herb garden modelled on that of the popular literary character, Brother Cadfael of Shrewsbury Abbey.

Theriacs and Christ

The King of Pontus, Mithridates VI, lived in fear of death by poisoning. He was an amateur pharmacist who devised an antidote to most poisons. This 'universal antidote', that contained tolerable doses of many poisons, was to be taken regularly to build up a specific immunity to lethal doses of its constituents — a very advanced concept for 111 BC! The final preparation contained 54 ingredients and was so effective that, when Mithridates really wanted to end his own life, he was unable to do so and had to command a slave to kill him! The preparation became known as *antidotum Mithridaticum* and a universal antidote to poison was also called a theriac.

Nero, who also lived in fear of death by poisoning, adopted Mithridates' antidote and ordered Andromachus, his Greek physician, to revise the formula. He added 20 more components and the 70 components were pulverized and reduced with honey to an *electuary* — a medicated paste prepared with honey. The name *therica Andromachi* has survived to this day. The new preparation owed its success to the increase in quantity of opium, as well as inclusion of the flesh of adders. When he presented it to Nero, it was accompanied by a poem beseeching Asclepius to increase its potency. Galen adopted the prescription and the poem, which were incorporated into his publication *de Antidotis*, Book *II* [28].

The theriac became symbolic of the supreme remedy, namely Christ. Artists depicting religious themes portrayed the theriac jar accompanied by an apple; the apple represented the original sin in the Garden of Eden and physical disease was regarded as a consequence of this. Artistic depictions of the apple and the theriac jar became symbolic of sin and disease, redemption, cure and salvation[28].

The potency and therapeutic spectrum of Christian pharmaceuticals were enhanced by the addition of religious symbols to the labelling. Pharmacy jars were decorated with symbols of Christ, the Virgin Mary or depictions of the healing saints.

Healing by touch
Healing by touch was part of the '*incubatio*' ritual in the *abaton* of Asclepius (Figure 37). Christ also healed many by his touch and subsequent Christian physicians continued the practice[37]. This gift was bestowed on Clovis I, King of the Franks, after his baptism on Christmas Day in 496 AD[38]. It became an hereditary gift of Christian kings and the custom of royalty healing by touch continued until the reign of the Hanoverian Georges. They declined the practice on the basis that they had not inherited sufficient original royal blood to possess this magical power. The king contributed towards the expenses of attending the ceremony by a gift of a coin which had been blessed at the altar (the coin was a silver penny during the reign of Edward I, 1272–1307). In later centuries, healing was restricted to treating scrofula (King's Evil or tuberculosis of the cervical lymph glands). This disease, which commonly occurred among children aged between two and 12 years, was subject to remissions and the king, rather than the patient's immune system, received credit for the apparent cure. As British royalty became more aesthetic, it avoided touching the necks of unwashed subjects by transferring the healing power to a special coin called the 'touch piece'. Touch pieces came in a number of designs. The most famous (and certainly the most popular with patients) was the gold 'angel' portraying St Michael slaying the dragon of disease[39]. These carried a variety of religious inscriptions, such as: 'By thy cross save us, O Christ, our redeemer'; 'This is the Lord's doing and it is marvellous to our eyes'; 'To God alone be the glory of cure'.

Henry VII was the first monarch to initiate formal presentation ceremonies for the 'touch piece'. The coin, suspended from a white satin ribbon, was placed around the patient's neck at an appropriate time in the religious ceremony. This gift was a royal token of reassurance for cure and served as a talisman against recurrence (Figure 76)[40]. Many patients were treated in this way; it is recorded that Charles II healed 92,107 patients, although there are no valid statistical records of the results he obtained. The English clergy felt that the gift was unique to their king and this might explain the meagre five assured cures out of 2,400 patients treated by King Louis XVI at Paris[40]! Treatment failures were attributed to lack of faith. The lexicographer Samuel Johnson was one of the last participants of the ceremony and the best-publicized failure. Perhaps this experience helped to develop his somewhat sarcastic personality; the actual coin gifted to him is in the British Museum collection.

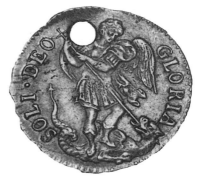

Figure 76 An especially minted gold 'touch piece' of Charles II (1662) which depicts St Michael slaying the dragon of disease. The coin is perforated for suspension around the neck (Photo from the TGH Drake Collection, courtesy Mrs Felicity Pope, Curator of the Canadian Museum of Health and Medicine, Toronto, ON, Canada)

Votives, talismans and reassurance

Christian churches and other places associated with healing continued the Asclepian tradition of votives and talismans. Christian 'healing shrines' are crowded with exhibits of crutches and other orthopaedic appliances left by pilgrims when their prayers were answered. Wax models of body parts and miniature metal plaques continue to decorate the sanctuaries of churches in Italy, Greece and other Mediterranean countries[41]. Many followers of Christ suspend a cross around their neck as a sign of faith and as a talisman. Christians, like the followers of Asclepius, also used coins as a talisman against disease. The most interesting Christian numismatic talismans are the *pesttalers* (plague dollars) of 16th century Germany, worn as a preventive against the plague and sold at places of pilgrimage. Some of these, especially those minted at Joachimstal and Schneeberg in Bohemia, were outstanding examples of medallic art[42–4]. These usually depicted Moses in the desert curing the children of Israel of their bites inflicted by the plague of fiery serpents. Moses, at God's command, had made a brass serpent and set it on a pole. Those who had been bitten looked at this and were cured. It is of interest that the Judaic pole had become Christianized and converted into a tau cross. These talismans were often inscribed with a biblical quotation from *Numbers* 21 (Figure 77) or some form of exhortation to repent one's sins. This holy icon parallels the 'pagan' practice of placing an image of Apollo with his bow and arrow above

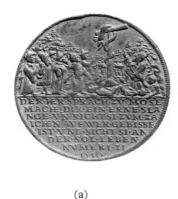
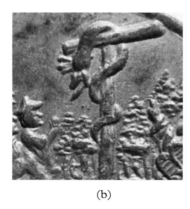

(a)   (b)

Figure 77

(a) A German *pesttaler* of 1530, depicting Moses and the brazen serpent encircling a T-shaped cross. The serpent and cross on the modern crest of the Royal Society of Medicine is identical to this and both are strikingly similar to the staff of Asclepius. Was this a Christian adaptation of the staff of Asclepius?

(b) Magnification of (a) showing the plague of serpents. These medals were usually pierced and hung around the neck as protection from the plague. This specimen remains in mint condition; perhaps the owner died before he had it pierced (Photo Ian Whan)

city gates as protection against epidemics and plague[1]. Unfortunately, neither device worked but, if actual Asclepian serpents had been placed in homes, meeting places and transportation vehicles, plague-transmitting rodents would have been eliminated and the outbreak contained!

In 1936, the Helpers League of the London Hospital made unique use of an Asclepian token in the 20th century. They minted a florin-sized silver-coloured token of health which depicted Hygieia on the obverse, standing clothed in a long skirt with shoulders covered, and was inscribed 'LONDON HOSPITAL' and 'HYGIEIA'. The reverse bore the legend 'HYGIEIA GODDESS OF HEALTH. CARRY YOUR TOKEN WITH YOU'. For this purpose, the tokens were frequently pierced for suspension around the neck[45]. Dr Gibbs reported that the tokens were sold for a shilling and an article in *The London Hospital Illustrated* 1936; **1**(5) described it with the headlines: 'Penny a month Helpers League; patients find easy way to help hospital they love'. It was claimed that, as a result of the tokens, 'Eastenders were rapidly becoming health conscious' and for this purpose, Hygieia, probably wisely, abandoned her snake[45].

Reassurance, an essential component of Asclepian temple medicine, was given to supplicants by an impressive statue of Asclepius and accompanying votives and testimonials. The church copied this by using the physical presence of the cross along with depictions of Jesus, Mary, the disciples and various saints. The bones or relics of a local saint were enshrined at healing centres throughout Christendom; votives, testimonials as well as discarded crutches and other invalid paraphernalia confirmed their healing powers. Silver anatomical thanks-offerings continue to be given and reverently displayed in the small church of the healing saints, Cosmas and Damian, located in the shadow of the Corinth acropolis which stands on the site of the Corinth Asclepieion.

During the reformation, many good-thinking Christians felt compelled to desecrate the traditions and places of worship of their brethren with the result that, in England today, saintly shrines have rarely survived. One is that of Edward the Confessor in Westminster Abbey and the other is in the Church of St Candida and Holy Cross at Whitchurch Canonicorum, Bridport, Dorset.

Hospices

Asclepian temples had often served as hospices and poorhouses. Following Constantine's adoption of Christianity, his mother, Helena, established a hospice dedicated to the care of the poor, downtrodden and chronically ill. This initiated a trend among ladies of the upper classes; the wealthy also donated funds to establish centres for palliative and spiritual care. Julian, the Apostate, believed these hospices were so popular among the masses that it would be necessary to re-establish similar pagan centres to facilitate the return to paganism. Recently, there has been a rebirth of the hospice, with increasing numbers of chronically ill patients receiving tender care in peaceful surroundings.

Dr Cecily Saunders initiated a trend when she re-established, in 1967, the ancient hospice principle with St Christopher's Hospice for the care of the terminally ill in London, England. Physical and psychosocial problems are addressed so patients may enjoy physical comfort as well as reassurance and peace in a pleasant, unregimented setting to live their last days to the fullest. With the aid of volunteers, the movement is spreading around the world and is offering hope and comfort to many patients with a variety of terminal diseases.

Christian religious healing in rural England

The shrine of St Wite in the church of St Candida and Holy Cross at Whitchurch Canonicorum, Dorset, illustrates the tradition of Christian religious healing. The intact tomb of St Wite rests on a platform in the

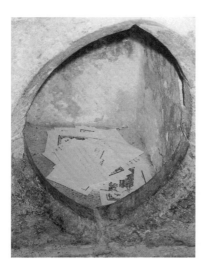

Figure 78 One of the three limb holes below the tomb of St Wite (Dorset, England) which continues to be used not only for limbs but also for the reception of written petitions seeking relief of illnesses and restoration of health (Photo GDH)

north transept of the church. Three 'limb holes' are present below her shrine, enabling supplicants seeking cure to place their diseased part in closer proximity to the bones of the saint. Her spiritual healing powers were also transferred to handkerchiefs that could be taken to those too ill to undertake a pilgrimage. Lepers, who were isolated from the congregation, were able to participate in her ritual healing by means of openings in the outer church wall behind the shrine.

Whenever a pilgrim had been cured in the past, he or she would cry out: 'Measure me for St Wite'. The diseased part of the body was measured and a candle of that size was made and given as a votive of thanks. If the recovered part was a hand or foot, the resultant candle would not be very large. However, in the case of the whole body, it was usual to wind the wick into a coil or 'trindle' before coating it with wax[46,47]. Discarded crutches, sticks and bandages were placed around the shrine and cured supplicants donated votive arms, legs and eyes that were displayed in a fashion similar to the votives at Asclepian temples. The healing tradition continues today—limb holes contain numerous petitions written on pre-printed postcards. Supplicants or their relatives and friends, along with their prayers, deposit the 'petitions' to St Wite; these are a modern counterpart to the votives used at Asclepian temples to attract his attention to the affliction (Figure 78).

A short distance away from the church is St Wite's well whose water, as late as the 1930s, had a reputation for being a sovereign cure for the eyes, reminiscent of the waters of Pergamum. At nearby Stonebarrow Hill, the wild periwinkles that grow in springtime are called St Candida's Eyes. This plant was introduced into Britain by the Romans and was used as both an astringent and remedy for chest diseases. Recently, its healing powers were rediscovered and one variety, *Vinca rosea* (Linn), is the source of the Vinca alkaloids considered as some of the best chemotherapy agents for treating certain leukaemias and malignant lymphomas.

The shrine of St Wite is located in an ancient church where the plinth of a Norman column has sunk below the floor level and is decorated by a Saxon carving of two roses on the wall of the nave and a Viking axe on the church tower. This spiritual place used the healing traditions of Asclepius and Hygieia with those of the healing saints.

Summary

In Greek and Roman times, the mystery and spiritual aspects of healing became allied to medical progress. Christianity adopted many of the same basic religious beliefs but they took precedence over whatever medical treatment was available.

Notes and references

1. Lane Fox R. *Pagans and Christians*. Middlesex: Penguin Books Ltd, 1985. This book reviews the pagan origins of Christian rituals which include: praying to the east; seasonal rituals; religious plays, holidays and processions; the rationalization of texts of the oracles; angels and visions; baptism and other practices.

2. New scientific technology is being developed for visualization of structures under standing buildings. This will offer great potential for further archaeological discoveries under the churches and cathedrals built over pagan temples in the centre of the towns of Roman Britain.

3. Parish church of Saint John the Baptist, Tunstall, Lancashire, England. See chapter 7: Aesculapius goes to Britain.

4. Whitman WB. Rome's Tiber island. *MD* December 1992: 25–9.

5. *AA essential explorer: ROME*. Basingstoke: AA Publishing, 1993.

6. Kerenyi C. *Asklepios*. Bolligen series LXV 3. New York: Pantheon Books, 1959.

7. The island was also associated with the Jewish community who opened the first Jewish hospital in Rome in 1880. This structure now provides an outpatient geriatric service. 'Fatebenefratelli' enjoys a good relationship with the Jewish community; during World War Two, many residents of the nearby ghetto were confined to their hospital beds with plaster on their legs which prevented them from being transported.

8. In the 18th century, another beneficent religious order was located on the island: the devotees of Jesus at Calvary, or the 'Red Hoods', specialized in retrieving bodies of suicide victims from the Tiber so they could have a Christian burial.

9. The jongleurs were a well-known class in medieval society. They earned their living as public entertainers by telling tales of epic heroes, singing and playing the harp or viola, tumbling, juggling or leading dancing bears. Some were attached to the households of great nobles; others, like Rahere, went from place to place and were rewarded by gifts or money[10].

10. Whitteridge G, Stokes V. *The Royal Hospital of St Bartholomew, London*. London: The Governors of the Hospital of St Bartholomew, 1961.

11. Burrage C. Personal view (St Bartholomew's Hospital). *BMJ* 1984; **288**: 143.

12. The campaign was conducted not only by people from around the world whose lives had been touched by St Bart's, but also on the pavement outside a volunteer group carried the message to passers-by under the shadow of a colossal effigy of Rahere.

13. Edelstein EJ, Edelstein L. *Asclepius, a collection and interpretation of the Testimonies. Volume 2.* Baltimore: Johns Hopkins Press, 1945: 194–5 (footnotes).
14. Nilsson MP. Divine service in late antiquity. *The Harvard theological review* 1945; **38**: 63.
15. Kroll J. *Die Antike* 1926: **2**: 258. Christians enjoyed a heritage from the Hebrews and this may have influenced the singing component of their services.
16. The original sanctuary knocker is preserved in the Durham cathedral treasury.
17. During the 1930s Great Depression in the US, the re-election of President Roosevelt and his New Deal election platform were characterized by the song 'Happy days are here again'.
18. Sherrard P, Editors of TIME-LIFE Books. *Byzantium: the great ages of man.* New York: Time Inc, 1966.
19. *CNR* Spring 1995; **20–1**: 20–116 (Sear, Byzantine coins, 1800; DOC III 6a).
20. *Classical coins.* CNG 1995; **33**: 1434.
21. *CNR* 1994; **19**(4): 446.
22. English coins have either portrayed a cross or arranged crests in the form of a cross since the reign of King Ecgberht (732–66 AD). The penny began with a small cross that expanded in 1016 AD to occupy the reverse of the coin (long cross penny). This decreased in size during the reign of Edward the Confessor (1042–66) (short cross penny). It then underwent further reductions in size, the cross ceasing to be shown on pennies after the Commonwealth Period (1649–60). A small cross was re-introduced by Queen Elizabeth II but disappeared in 1968 with the introduction of new pence and the decimal currency, which were minted in 1968 but dated 1971.
23. Berman A. *Papal numismatic history. The Emancipation of the Papal state.* 2nd edn. New York: Attic Books Ltd, 1991.
24. Malloy AG, Preston FP, Seltman AJ. *Coins of the crusader states.* New York: Attic Books Ltd, 1994.
25. Jacob K. *Coins and Christianity.* 2nd edn. London: Seaby, 1985.
26. Yeoman RS. *Moneys of the Bible.* Wisconsin: Whitman Publishing Company, 1961.
27. Hendin D. *Guide to Biblical coins.* 3rd edn. New York: Amphora Nyack, 1996.
28. Schouten J. *The rod and serpent of Asklepios.* London: Elsever Publishing Company, 1967: 73.
29. The miracle would be impossible today. The Ethiopian would have to sign a donor consent form before death giving his permission to donate his leg for transplantation. Without this, his family would sue and human rights organizations would protest the choice of donor.
30. Lyons AS, Petrucelli RJ. *Medicine: an illustrated history.* New York: Harry N Abrams Inc, 1978.
31. Dewhurst J. Cosmas and Damian, patron saints of doctors. *Lancet* 1988; **2**: 1479–80.
32. Gerlitt J. Cosmas and Damian, the patron saints of physicians. *Ciba Symposia* 1939; **1**(4):118–21.
33. Pamphlet published by the Royal Society of Medicine: *The history and evolution of the Royal Society of Medicine*; section on the Coat of Arms.
34. Hart GD. English token coins and medicine. *Can Med Assoc J* 1966; **95**: 1311–7.
35. Frey FF. Saints in medical history. *Clio Medica* 1979; **14**(1): 35–70.
36. Cohen RA, Down K. St Apollonia in Britain. *Br Dental J* 1989; **166**(5): 181–2.
37. Christ and his disciples healed many by touch. See: *Mark* 6:5; 7:32; 16:18. *Luke* 4:40; 13:13. *Acts* 28:8.

38. Harrup A. Touch pieces: coins and medals. *Ciba Symposia*, 1968.

39. An 'angel' was the standard doctor's fee and represented the cost of living for three days.

40. Spaulding M, Welch P. *Nurturing yesterday's child: a portrayal of the Drake Collection of pediatric history*. Toronto: Natural Heritage/Natural History Inc, 1994.

41. Gerlitt J. Votive offerings. *Ciba Symposia* 1939; **1**(4): 122–5.

42. In ancient times, 'plague' (*pestilentia*) meant contagious disease with high mortality and included bubonic plague as well as smallpox, cholera, yellow fever, malaria and other communicable diseases. Kirsh B. Plague and coins. *Ciba Symposia 9* 1948; **10**: 107–9.

43. Brettauer J. Katalog der sammlung. *Medicina in nummis*. Wien: Pesttaler und Pestmedaillen, 1937: 110–8.

44. Pfeiffer, Rutland. Die deutscher pestamulete. *Pestilentia in nummis*. Tübingen, 1882.

45. Gibbs D. *Emblems, tokens and tickets of the London Hospital (1740–1985) and the London Hospital Medical College (1785–1985)*. London: Gibbs D, 1985.

46. Waters C. *Who was St Wite? The Saint of Whitchurch Canonicorum*. Dorset: Waters C, 1980.

47. Creed S. *The church of St Candida (St Wite) and Holy Cross*. Sherborne: Dorset Western Vale Publishing, 1987.

Chapter 12

Asclepius and medical practice today

Doctors have inherited many traditions from Hippocratic physicians and their Roman successors. Ethical guidelines and clinical methods of the Hippocratic school are still followed; they review their research results in a philosophical fashion and, like their Greek and Roman antecedents, continue the search for new medicines from the plant and animal kingdom. They perform surgery with instruments similar to those developed by the Greek and Roman physicians and are re-assessing the ancient tradition of healing by touch. The concept of a healthcare team continues but, although not based in heaven, it is more diverse and very temporal. The serpent-entwined staff of Asclepius remains the logo of the physician.

Oath of Hippocrates

The oath of Hippocrates is the most important document in the historical archive of medicine. Although the oldest surviving fragment is from an Egyptian papyrus of around 300 AD, classical scholars have been able to use a variety of sources to reconstruct the original text of c400 BC. It is believed that Hippocrates was not the author, but was written by an unknown practitioner from the Hippocratic school[1,2]. The contents have been modified to adapt to the changing demographics of time. Even the gods to whom it was sworn have been altered or allied with other deities so as to comply with the beliefs of physicians from Christian, Islamic and other faiths: 'God the One and Three, the father of Hygieia and Panacea' (several Christian versions also emphasized its adopted holiness by transcribing the words in the form of a cross). The Arabic oath preceded the invocation to Asclepius with: 'Allah the master of life and death, the giver of health, and the creator of healing and every treatment'.

An enigma surrounds the oath, as it is not known who took it and under what circumstances it was sworn. Lack of regular use is emphasized by the absence of its reference by classical writers. Scribonius Largus, the ancient authority on pharmacology, regretted the deficiency of moral rules, medical directives and compulsory oaths. Galen did not mention the oath in his writings but referred his readers to Hippocratic texts for guidance on ethics and medical conduct. The 20th century historian, Ludwig Edelstein, felt that in ancient times most Greek and Roman physicians neither took the oath nor followed its ethical directives. Professor Vivian Nutton stated in 1995 that tracing the history of the taking of the oath was an extraordinarily difficult task. 'Evidence shows that the oath was an option taken by a minority in one place at one time and was never imposed by law or custom, neither in pagan Greece and Rome, nor in the Muslim world, nor in medieval Europe.'[3] The earliest-known university use was not at student level but was applied for administrative purposes at Wittenberg in 1508; the earliest obligatory student or graduate participation did not occur until 1804 at Montpellier[3]. It was adopted enthusiastically in the US between 1840 and 1860, but this interest declined; apart from the initiation ceremony of the Alpha Omega Alpha (AOA) Honour Medical Society, founded in 1906 in the US, undergraduate swearing of the oath was not taken seriously in the first half of the 20th century. Students, myself included, did not understand the depth of its significance and regarded taking such an anachronistic oath as a focus on traditions and hindrance to the exciting opportunities of medical progress. In the 1960s, however, there was a renaissance of interest in morality and ethics, including the swearing of the oath by medical schools in the western world.

The following is the benchmark translation of the original Hippocratic oath used by Ludwig Edelstein in the *Bulletin of the History of Medicine* in 1943 (© The Johns Hopkins University Press):

'I swear by Apollo Physician and Asclepius and Hygieia and Panaceia and all the gods and goddesses, making them my witnesses, that I will fulfil according to my ability and judgment this oath and this covenant:

To hold him who has taught me this art as equal to my parents and to live my life in partnership with him, and if he is in need of money to give him a share of mine, and to regard his offspring as equal to my brothers in male lineage and to teach them this art — if they desire to learn it — without fee and covenant; to give a share of precepts and oral instruction and all the other learning to my sons and to the sons of him who has instructed me and to pupils who have signed the covenant and have taken an oath according to the medical law, but to no one else.

I will apply dietetic measures for the benefit of the sick according to my ability and judgment; I will keep them from harm and injustice. I will neither give a deadly drug to anybody if asked for it, nor will I make a suggestion to this effect. Similarly I will not give to a woman an abortive remedy. In purity and holiness I will guard my life and my art. I will not use the knife, not even on sufferers from stone, but will withdraw in favor of such men as are engaged in this work. Whatever houses I may visit, I will come for the benefit of the sick, remaining free of all intentional injustice, of all mischief and in particular of sexual relations with both female and male persons, be they free or slaves. What I may see or hear in the course of the treatment or even outside of the treatment in regard to the life of men, which on no account one must spread abroad, I will keep to myself holding such things shameful to be spoken about.

If I fulfil this oath and do not violate it, may it be granted to me to enjoy life and art, being honored with fame among all men for all time to come; if I transgress it and swear falsely, may the opposite of all this be my lot.'[4] Hippocrates *Ius Iurandum, 1* (sworn oath)

Edelstein's original translation has been divided into four paragraphs to emphasize its four separate components. The invocation to the gods and the continuity with classical medicine, as mentioned in the first paragraph, has already been discussed. The second paragraph describes the relationship of a student or apprentice with his teacher, and his vow to fulfil 'family' obligations to him and continue his tradition of teaching. If there was a medical school at Cos in 400 BC, and if the author of the oath was an experienced clinician, then there is a strong possibility that the oath was originally intended to be taken by a new graduate before beginning medical practice. This hypothesis must be examined through the contemporary eyes of a student at Cos at that time. The hypothetical student would believe that he is swearing the oath to the gods he worships and whose depictions and activities form part of his daily life. After becoming a doctor, the novitiate physician would join the divine healthcare team and become a surrogate son of Asclepius. Previous work by Nutton has established the limited use of the oath in ancient times[3]. We must concentrate on Cos for evidence to support a hypothesis for student use of the oath in ancient times. Hippocrates' *Epistulae* II (ET 568) has a suggestive reference: ' . . . and the taking up of the staff happened to be celebrated on that day [annual festival of the Asclepiads] and the annual festival, as you know, a solemn festival for us [people of Cos], and a magnificent procession to the cypress grove, which it was customary to be led by those who were related to the god'. This quotation comes from a letter Hippocrates was reputed to have written to his friend in Abdera. It is said to be one from a series relating to a petition

Hippocrates received from this city in northern Greece (Thrace)[5]. His letter described the visit of a mutual acquaintance to Cos but does not elaborate on details of the festival; quite possibly, he presupposes that his acquaintance is familiar with the circumstances.

Was the solemn festival the occasion for the taking of an oath by a novitiate physician (graduate) about to become a surrogate son of Asclepius, and who had to swear an oath to the members of the divine healthcare team? Was the sacred cypress grove an appropriate place for such a ceremony? Was a staff symbolic of Asclepius given to a new graduate? The setting and ceremony described seems ideal for performance of an equivalent to a modern graduation ceremony. This possibility merits mention beside Montpellier as the first place where a student took an ethical oath for medicine.

The third paragraph of the oath outlines general rules of treatment, basic standards of medical practice and the physician's obligation to patients. The commitment to apply dietary measures in prime position is of great interest and doctors should still follow this. Many of today's health problems, especially heart and cardiovascular disease, could be prevented, treated and improved by eliminating intake of chips (excess of harmful fats), cigarette smoking (intake of substance abuse) and 'couch potatoes' (inadequate exercise with constant eating of snacks). This paragraph also contains the original guideline of ethical behaviour for the ideal physician; its principles remain a universal consensus with 'timeless validity', accepted by all ethical medical practitioners. Ludwig Edelstein analysed the ethics contained in this paragraph and concluded that a physician who had studied the medical teachings of Pythagoras had written it[4].

The fourth paragraph emphasizes the sincerity of the declaration.

Pythagorean theories

Pythagorean theories contained the Hippocratic oath. They believed that all ingested food and drink created a certain disposition of the soul, and that harm and injustice resulted from gluttony. They felt excess satiation of appetites caused an imbalance between body and soul that caused illness. Pythagorean thinking may have been based on observations that some of the local population suffered severe reactions to the ingestion of fava beans. They emphasized the importance of treatment by diet and used medications to purify the body, and music to purify the soul.

Pythagoreans believed in the sanctity of life and considered killing to be a sin. To them, the embryo was an animate being from the moment of conception, which was the only justification for coitus. Their beliefs were unique in the ancient world and they were the only group to completely ban abortion. They prohibited the giving of drugs that could assist suicide or were for the purpose of poisoning. Pythagorean physicians opposed surgical treatment and relegated it to those engaged in the practice. They opposed all forms of licentious behaviour and sexual indiscretions. They also believed in confidentiality in all matters and maintained the privacy of their own philosophy.

Continuity of the oath
The tradition of clinical teaching has continued. Undergraduate and postgraduate medical students today are taught voluntarily and without stipend — many universities, including the University of Toronto, continue this custom. Students still bond to their teachers and adopt them as role models, father figures and lifetime advisors.

Physicians remain concerned with diet and frequently state that the patient is what he eats. Regulation of diet is an essential component of therapy for a variety of today's diseases, such as: obesity, hypertension, heart disease, diabetes, constipation, spastic colon, ulcers, liver disease, gout and neurological disorders. Proper nutrition is advised as a prophylaxis against sickness in infancy, childhood, adolescence, adulthood, pregnancy and old age; nutritional assessment is an important element in preventing postoperative morbidity and mortality.

Present-day physicians, like the Pythagoreans, prohibit ingestion of the fava bean to patients with glucose 6 phosphate dehydrogenase (G6PD) enzyme deficiency. This enzyme deficiency is a hereditary condition rendering the red blood cells susceptible to destruction by a variety of agents. The fava bean is one such agent and its ingestion causes explosive destruction of red blood cells (haemolysis). The resulting acute haemolytic anaemia produces profound symptoms and such episodes may be fatal. Today, the highest incidence of this condition occurs in southern Italy, in the area of Pythagoras and his followers.

Doctors continue to protect patients from harm and injustice when they actively intervene on their behalf with government agencies, insurance companies, as well as in a variety of medico-legal situations where they are obliged to supply, within reasonable time, a medico-legal report. They also continue to refuse to dispense a deadly drug, although opinions are divided on the ethics of physician-assisted suicide and euthanasia. Until recently, abortion was performed only for specific medical indications and no patient could receive it on demand. 'Freedom of choice' has now entered the medical scene but abortion is still not universally accepted or available — many physicians continue to believe the embryo is an animate being.

Doctors 'guard their art in purity and holiness' when they serve at their own expense and risk in underdeveloped countries of the world.

The prohibition of using the knife has posed a problem to some of those studying the oath, as this dictum is not mentioned elsewhere in *The Hippocratic corpus*. It has been suggested that this was a prohibition applied only to those not fully qualified or that a teacher considered this task beneath his dignity. Christian attitudes against surgery in general have also been mentioned. Perhaps the academics raising the question have been searching for something beyond their experience. Many doctors do not perform surgery and leave it to those who have special training. Even today, a neurosurgeon or cardiovascular surgeon will not remove a bladder stone, continuing to 'withdraw in favour of such men as are engaged in this work'!

Updating the Hippocratic oath and new guidelines for medical practice

Recent scientific advances and social changes have necessitated continuing expansion of the basic guidelines of the Hippocratic oath. New guides to the ethical behaviour of physicians have been created to address issues resulting from transplant technology, gene therapy, in vitro fertilization, controlled clinical trials, human experimentation, cloning and other advances. Patients and relatives now demand open and frank disclosure of medical information and no longer enjoy a paternalistic relationship with their physician. Treatment now requires informed patient consent and doctors must respect a patient's rights. Doctors must be accountable to a patient's family, hospital administrators, insurance companies, government agencies and global budgets. The growth of a litigation-conscious society has stimulated the practice of defensive medicine.

Medical ethicists and professional healthcare administrators demand written mission statements describing purpose, responsibility, accountability and basic acceptable standards of medical practice from individual physicians, hospitals and university departments.

Some of the new guidelines acknowledge the basic contribution of the Hippocratic oath to the field. 'Whatever houses I may visit, I will come for the benefit of the sick, remaining free of all intentional injustice...' was a statement of the physician's obligation to the patient that remains the foundation of the Canadian Medical Association Code of Ethics. The rapid pace of societal changes and advances in medical practice have made it necessary for a 1996 revision to the code established in 1990[6,7].

Confidentiality of patient information remains sacrosanct and doctors consider their medical records confidential. Patient permission must be obtained before disclosing any details to a third party. Disclosure of patient health details to lawyers and insurance companies needs signed patient permission — a written patient request is even necessary for the transfer of the medical record to another physician. However, in Canada under certain circumstances, physicians must provide information to protect society, such as when the patient is unfit to drive. In 1998, the Ontario College of Physicians and Surgeons adopted the principle that physicians have a duty to divulge confidential information when a patient reveals a plausible intention to do serious harm to a third party[8].

Medical disciplinary bodies have zero tolerance for any action suggestive of a sexual advance towards a patient or a member of his/her household; transgression of this trust results in suspension with disgrace. Physicians continue to be honoured among men and their credibility with society ranks above all professions and occupations. Today, physicians are liable to lose their licence and face public disgrace if they 'transgress' from the very same covenants undertaken by those who swore the oath of Hippocrates.

In 1997, the World Medical Association (WMA) planned to update the ethics contained in the 1948 Declaration of Geneva. At that time, it asked the British Medical Association (BMA) to prepare a draft update of the oath of Hippocrates. The BMA revision integrated into new wording the mutually shared values of ethical codes of practice from worldwide sources; the text aimed to be a politically correct, unifying force, superseding national, ethnic, religious and cultural boundaries. The BMA felt that 'the value of this update will be all the greater if it comes into use by every doctor qualifying from every medical school in the world'[9]. Despite this, WMA committees were unable to agree on a consensus and the project has been cancelled [personal communication: BMA, June 1999].

The great expansion in medical progress has been accompanied by societal changes with the emergence of new ethical considerations for the practice of medicine. These are not valid reasons to abandon the traditional sheet anchor of medical ethics. The original oath of Hippocrates requires pruning of items not pertinent to the present and should be accompanied by an addendum detailing the expanding advances of medical practice. Remove the pantheism of the invocation and swear to Asclepius alone. Remove the section dealing with teaching of medicine in antiquity. Translate into concise language the original guiding ethical concepts, as well as the rewards of medical practice and punishments of malpractice. This edited format would offer continuity with the past and comprehension for the present. It would be the starting point for the growing spectrum of medical ethics detailed in an accompanying addendum. The swearing of the oath need not be obligatory, but the facility for students and practitioners to do so should be available — their participation would be encouraged by issuing a certificate authenticating their solemn acceptance of the established principles of medical ethics.

Hippocratic approach

The Hippocratic approach continues to influence medical practice: 'The physician must be able to tell what has gone on before [past history], to know the present [history of present illness], and to suggest a prognosis ... with two particular intentions in mind regarding diseases, to do good or to do no harm'[10,11].

Whenever my colleague, Professor Peter Fitzpatrick, and I made a decision after a 'combined consultation' for palliative cancer therapy, we followed the Hippocratic dictum of 'if you can't do any good then don't do any harm'. Although we trained 3,500 miles apart, we both had teachers who followed Hippocratic teachings and, therefore, inherited a common philosophy of care: 'The art [of healing] comprises three elements: the disease, the patient and the physician. The physician is the servant of the art. The patient must cooperate with the physician in fighting the disease'[11]. 'The disease, the patient and the physician' summarizes current medical philosophy. Patients are now participating in decisions regarding therapy, and those who are motivated for cure do better than those with a negative attitude.

The Hippocratic text, *Aphorisms*, contains succinct statements about life, death and disease; the first and best known of these summarized the challenges of research and medical practice: 'Life is short, art is long; opportunities are short-lived, experimentation is risky, judgement is fraught with difficulties. Not only must the physician be ready to do what is necessary, but the patient and also those in attendance must play their part as well and the external factors must be right'[12]. Art is indeed long; in fact, a generation of additional research was needed to advance from successful tissue culture of bone marrow cells in the laboratory to a practical technique for human bone marrow transplantation. Success is elusive as experiments in the laboratory are adversely affected by a host of external factors. Recognition of the potential for experiments to be dangerous has led to the establishment of ethics and human experimentation committees to monitor research programmes in hospitals and universities. Hippocrates foresaw the difficulties of research; today, the accurate interpretation of research needs judgement by peer review of a written or spoken presentation. In addition to authenticating the study, discussion following the presentation helps philosophical analysis and creates suggestions for further study and application. This academic route of research recalls the observation of Aristotle that one might begin with philosophy but would end with medicine, or start with medicine and find oneself in philosophy.

The Hippocratic treatise entitled *Law* stated: 'Inexperience, on the other hand, is a bad treasure and a bad storehouse for those who possess it ... it nurtures both cowardice and rashness. For cowardliness suggests a lack of powers and rashness a lack of skill'[13]. Today's medical student studies medical ethics and is urged to understand basic medico-legal issues. If students were to learn one thing about practising defensive medicine, then these words, written before the days of litigation, would be worth remembering.

The clinical approach of the Hippocratic school continues today — good physicians still listen carefully to the patient's description of symptoms and record details of their onset and progress. Overall, patient management includes attention to variations of age, diet, occupation, residence, family history, religious and ethnic factors. Physicians continue to begin their written record with a thumbnail description of the patient, which frequently records the facial expression; the term '*Hippocratic facies*' continues to be used to describe the portent of imminent death.

In ancient Greece, malaria and pneumonia were common causes of illness and mortality. Hippocratic physicians recorded meticulously the degree and cycles of fever: 'When in a state of continuous fever, breathing difficulties occur and also delirium, death cannot be far away'[14]. They paid particular attention to findings of their physical examination of the abdomen; their descriptions of the spleen recorded in *The Hippocratic corpus* challenge the modern clinical reader with diagnostic possibilities, such as chronic enlargement of the spleen and splenic infarct.

After obtaining a complete patient history and performing an accurate physical examination, a physician combines these facts with his past experience and learning to deduce a differential diagnosis of the likely causes of illness and to formulate a working provisional diagnosis for the illness. In addition, from past experience with similar cases, the doctor may be able to give the prognosis. The doctor's follow-up notes of the patient and illness should describe the treatment given, the patient's progress through illness, its outcome and any complications. Record of this information may serve as a basis for future teaching and research. Hippocratic 'case reports' undoubtedly contributed to the various general medical adages and aphorisms of the Hippocratic school. Reality of the Hippocratic method has been confirmed by two recent, retrospective clinical reviews. In 1992, Peterson, Holbrook and Hales studied previously undiagnosed medical conditions and demonstrated that an accurate and detailed history of an illness alone gave a diagnosis in 76% of cases; physical examination alone allowed diagnosis in 12%, as did laboratory tests[15]. A further review by Bordage, in 1995, revealed a recent trend away from patient history and physical examination towards greater reliance being placed on laboratory tests. This new, computerized approach was found to be less cost-effective than the traditional reliance on the age-old approach of the Hippocratic school[16,17]. Incredible as it seems, an experienced physician of today using the methods of the Hippocratic school is able to diagnose 88% of cardiac, pulmonary, gastrointestinal and certain other diseases.

Quality medical records of today continue in the Hippocratic school style and are the source of medical rounds, case reviews, medical audits, quality control and retrospective clinical research. They are the benchmark for assessing the quality of patient care and are used by medical peer review committees to assess hospital accreditation and individual medical competence.

From Galen to Glaxo[18]
Pharmaceutical accomplishments of Greek and Roman physicians are discussed in chapter 8. The books of Scribonius Largus (*Compositones* 43–8 AD), Dioscorides (*de Materia medica* 77 AD) and Galen (*de Compositione medicamentorum* c175 AD) were preserved by scholars and scribes of Byzantium and the monasteries — their texts continued to be standard references on pharmacology until the 17th century. At that time, advances in the knowledge of chemistry led to new techniques of analysis applicable to herbs, plants, minerals, animal substances and preparations used in folk medicine. The knowledge and principles of ancient physicians were expanded and foundations for the accuracy and spectrum of modern pharmacy were laid.

Renaissance pharmacists, like Dioscorides and Scribonius Largus before them, took their interests in native remedies and local plants on voyages of exploration. When the crew of Jacques Cartier, the first French explorer in New France (Canada) in 1535, suffered from scurvy, it was discovered that the native people treated this condition with an infusion made from the leaves and bark of a tree[19]. In 1605,

Sieur de Monts established his first colony at Port Royal (Nova Scotia) and appointed an apothecary from Paris — Louis Hébert[20] — to look after the health of the colony. Hébert established a herb garden and learned the medical treatments used by the local Micmac Indians[21]. One such remedy was *Hydrastis canadensis* (goldenseal) that was used for treating wounds, ulcers and vaginitis. The preparation became so popular with subsequent European settlers that the plant was overpicked and nearly became extinct — just like the silphium plant from ancient Cyrenaica[22,23]!

The monastic belief that plants drew the cure of disease from God's earth was brought to the North American colonies. In 1774, the Shaker sect, most notable of the Protestant sectarians, began cultivating medicinal plants at New Lebanon, New York. They started a herb business in 1800 and, by the end of the 19th century, were collecting herbs and roots from more than 248 varieties of plants. Their products, which sold internationally to apothecaries and physicians, were renowned for purity and reliability. Many of these, such as hyoscyamus, belladonna, poppy, dock and horehound, were familiar to the Asclepiads and are still used today[21].

In the late 18th century, European colonists and explorers in South America became aware of the value of Peruvian barks for alleviation of malaria symptoms and other intermittent fevers. In 1817, intensive pharmaceutical investigation led to the isolation by the French pharmacologists, Pierre Joseph Pelletier and Joseph Bienaimé Caventou, of the alkaloid emetine from ipecacuanha (ipecac root), strychnine and brucine from the ignacia bean (*Strychnos nux-vomica*) and quinine from red and yellow cinchona (Peruvian bark). Quinine continues to be one of the most economical drugs for treating and preventing malaria. Many other useful drugs have been discovered by laboratory analysis of 'local treatment traditions'. The most significant of these was the investigation of *Vinca rosea* (periwinkle) by Noble, Beer and Cutts in the Collip Medical Research Laboratory at the University of Western Ontario. This plant had been used for many decades as a family medicine for the treatment of diabetes mellitus; while investigating the anti-diabetic properties of this periwinkle, these researchers discovered a new plant alkaloid possessing major therapeutic value in the treatment of haematological malignancies[24,25].

The methods of Largus, Dioscorides and Galen continue today but are aided by sophisticated laboratory techniques. Broad-based screening programmes are applied to ethnobotany, botany, biology and microbiology in search of new compounds with potential therapeutic action[26]. The stocks of present-day pharmacies follow the recommendation of Scribonius Largus in his book *Parasceuasticon* (Regarding Preparations) that two to three proven compounds be prepared and ready at hand for each and every disease[27]. Research pharmacologists no longer trudge along the ancient *itinera* of the Roman empire but travel on the information highway to reach the same destination—better medicines for better health.

From sounds to sonic booms
The broad range of surgical instruments developed by Greek and Roman physicians facilitated many surgical procedures. Many of these instruments have been recovered by archaeologists and have been found in every part of the Roman world—this demonstrates their ready availability and widespread use. If a selection of such instruments were placed on a tray then, apart from being made from bronze, they would resemble a present-day tray of operating room instruments prepared for an abdominal operation.

Although ancient doctors did not have sophisticated knowledge of antisepsis, they did use the antiseptic properties of wine; the level of personal hygiene at the Roman *valetudinaria* certainly exceeded that of any hospital up to the latter half of the 19th century. Estimates for the incidence of postoperative infections in Roman times were probably biased by the horrendous statistics of the 19th century! Even Lord Lister, the inventor of modern day asepsis, said: 'Asepsis in this imperfect world is not to be trusted, human carelessness and fallibility are common'.

Despite limited formal anatomical knowledge in classical times, it was only after the advent of anaesthesia and blood transfusion that modern surgery began to expand the horizons for surgical cure. For instance, the extent and position of lesions are now visualized preoperatively via three-dimensional imaging and computer technology. Visualization of the operative field has been improved by the use of flexible fibre optics and dissecting microscopes. Microvascular techniques have advanced the potential of operative repair and isolation perfusion pumps have extended the time available for surgical procedures.

Stones previously located by palpation via a probe or sound are now visualized on three-dimensional computer screens and can be destroyed by the ultrasonic boom created from sound waves targeted on them. The Hippocratic oath presaged the techniques of lithotripsy when it suggested that the treatment of stone be left to 'such as are craftsmen therein'! Replacement joint surgery is enabling the lame to walk, and laser ophthalmology the blind to see. Many healing miracles of Asclepius and Christ are becoming daily surgical procedures, while transplant techniques are approaching the miracle operation of Sts Cosmas and Damian.

Healing by faith

Patients were treated at Asclepian temples by conservative therapy, concurrent medical care and 'incubation' in the *abaton*. The incubation treatment involved a combination of healing by faith, spirit and touch. Christianity continued a similar tradition of healing but emphasized the need for faith. Although spiritual healing methods have not been accepted by scientific medicine, they survive in the present-day world. In 1986, the BMA reviewed evidence for the value of spiritual healing and concluded that its effects were psychological as 'healers' spent more time with their patients[28]. Their report did not stem the tide of resurgent interest in Britain, and the ethical rule book of the General Medical Council of Great Britain has been amended to allow doctors to delegate patient care to 'healers' and to allow general practitioners to employ them in their surgeries. The techniques of healing by faith are: faith healing in a purely religious context; spiritual healing or the laying on of hands; therapeutic touch; Reiki healing which involves the laying on of hands and distant healing techniques[29].

The increased awareness of spiritual healing has stimulated controlled, scientific research into the phenomenon. Hodges and Scofield, at the Department of Biological Sciences, Wye College, University of London, conducted studies with non-sensate targets which eliminated the possibility of a psychological effect[29]. Their controlled study used a 'gifted healer' and their 'diseased' organism was salt-stressed cress seed; experiments, which were repeated six times, showed the healer was capable of stimulating seed recovery and growth at a high level of statistical significance in five of the tests. Other authors have reported statistically significant results with additional non-sensate experiments, such as human red blood cells and platelets, as well as bacteria and fungi[29]. The mechanism for this action has not yet been identified, but it has been hypothesized that some form of energy, or spectrum of energies, exists that is undetectable by current scientific methods[30].

The review by Hodges and Scofield was published as a discussion paper in the *Journal of the Royal Society of Medicine*[29] and will no doubt generate a great deal of discussion. This reflects the catholic interests represented within medical care and it is reassuring that the 'high tech' world of today's medicine can pause and assess such simple procedures. If research is able to establish objective scientific validity for the technique of 'spiritual healing', there is potential to decrease present healthcare costs. Such validity could even establish a scientific basis for the soundness of Asclepius' and Christ's reported cures. It would also necessitate governing bodies of physicians to reassess their attitudes about touching the patient[31].

The healthcare team

Asclepian temple medicine used many assistants — also the miraculous cures usually involved a serpent, dog or temple priest. Patients could also consult Hygieia, Telesphorus, Panacea, Machaon, Podalirius, Apollo, Chiron and others. The Asclepiads called on the services of the associated gods, as well as practitioners more experienced with pharmacy and surgery, and assistance by their apprentices and paramedical personnel. Medical care continues as a team effort but the size of the team varies with the complexities of the case. A major organ transplant may involve the collaboration and skills of at least 100 professional personnel.

Staff of Asclepius

The single, serpent-entwined staff of Asclepius has been the symbol of healthcare providers for more than 2,500 years (Figure 24)[32]. After the Roman empire became Christian, Christ and his saints replaced Asclepius as the supreme healer and the canonized physicians, Cosmas and Damian, became the divine symbols of healthcare. Despite historical events, the role of Asclepius was not eradicated; his memory was preserved in ancient texts and monuments which, by serendipity and perhaps ironically, were facilitated by scriptoria of the monasteries and art collections of the church. Scholars of the Renaissance revived Asclepius from his state of suspended animation and he regained his role as the legendary supreme medical authority. At the time of the Reformation, the icons of Sts Cosmas and Damian were deliberately replaced by the staff and serpent of Asclepius which, once again, became the official symbol of medicine. However, at this time, the caduceus acquired a distinct role with pharmacology, chemistry and physics and it also became part of the official regalia of the Royal College of Physicians of London. These events contributed to a misconception that the caduceus, like the staff of Asclepius, is a medical symbol.

The caduceus assigned

The word 'caduceus' is akin to *kerykeion*, the ancient Greek for a herald's staff and a sign of peace. The symbol comprises two serpents

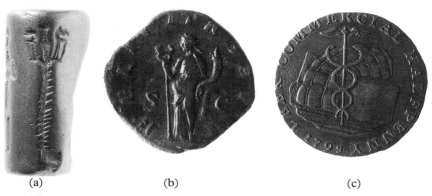

(a)   (b)   (c)

Figure 79
(a) Ancient Babylonian caduceus (c3000–2000 BC) used as a symbol of supreme sex (GDH)
(b) Caduceus portrayed on a third century AD Roman coin depicting the personification of Felicitas (GDH)
(c) Caduceus representing trade and commerce on an English token coin of 1793 (GDH)

facing each other at the upper end of a staff about which their bodies are entwined. With use, the finial of the staff acquired many variations including: a pair of wings, a pine cone, a mirror or a disc. The archaic form of the staff did not possess a pair of serpents but, in their place, there was a terminal figure 8 open at the top or a mirror image pair of threes (Figure 79).

More than 5,000 years ago, Mesopotamian farmers used a caduceus with two entwined serpents rising from the ground as their symbol for the life force responsible for crop regeneration. The Babylonian god, Ningizzida, used a staff surmounted by a serpent with externally facing twin-heads; this god was responsible for fertility in the spring and in the marriage bed, and was also responsible for bringing fevers and pestilence. About 4,000 years ago, a caduceus was used as a mace symbol for Ishtar, the Babylonian god of healing; in Graeco-Roman times, it became symbolic mainly of Hermes (Mercury) although it was also associated with other deities[33]. Some historians have argued that there was an evolutionary change from the Mesopotamian format of a twin-headed serpent surmounting the staff to the form of a staff entwined by serpents used by Hermes. However, Professor Friedlander, in his book *The golden wand of medicine*, reviewed all arguments for the evolution theory and concluded that there was currently not enough evidence for its confirmation[34].

Hermes' role with mankind varied at different times and places. He was mainly recognized as messenger of the gods and as peacemaker. He was patron of athletes and physical activity and performed additional roles such as: patron of trade and commerce, communication and interpretation skills (hermeneutics). He had many minor medical activities such as: relief of plagues, treatment of ailments of the lower extremities and the power to charm the eyes of men. He also had the dubious role of conducting dead souls to the underworld. He acquired many undesirable traits and was noted for dishonour, thievery as well as lascivious and promiscuous activities. Twelve other classical gods were associated with the caduceus (some of which are mentioned in chapter 3) but there is no epigraphic, numismatic or archaeological evidence for the caduceus ever having had an association with Asclepius.

In the Middle Ages, the planet Mercury influenced astrology, astronomy and alchemy. Alchemists thought quicksilver (the liquid metal *mercuria philosphorum*) was the first principle of all matter and incorporated its symbol (the caduceus) into their heraldic crests. They founded the principles of inorganic chemistry and pharmacy, and displayed the caduceus in the frontispiece of their text[35]. Physicians, who practised 'physic', used the fundamentals of alchemists and, as a result, had a legitimate association with the caduceus.

In 1556, the president of the Royal College of Physicians in London, John Caius, presented a silver wand or caduceus to the College. He stated the silver rod indicated that the president ruled with gentleness and clemency and that the serpents signified prudent rule. Caius' caduceus was not a symbol of physicians but was designated as an ensign of honour for the president to carry to indicate his presence at meetings and comitia. This wand had the arms of the College at its head, which were supported by two pairs of facing serpents, ie two caducei[36,37]. The Royal College of Physicians has presented replicas of their caduceus to the Royal College of Physicians of Canada and the American College of Physicians whose presidents continue its traditional role from 16th century London.

In 1851, the hospital corps of the US army selected the caduceus to be a symbol worn by hospital stewards. This decision was made on the basis of indicating non-combatant personnel and was not a medical symbol — perhaps this was done so that the caduceus could be seen as the symbol for a messenger of peace[38,39]. The US Public Health Service adopted its use in 1871. In 1902, it acquired its first major medical role when it became the symbol of the medical department of the US army. This choice was based on a false premise that the caduceus had been used as a medical corps symbol by the military of several foreign powers, notably the English (contrary to this statement, medical officers of the British army adopted the staff of Asclepius in 1898). French army medical officers have used an Asclepian staff since 1798 and Prussian army medical officers began to use the staff of Asclepius in 1868. Before this, the French had contributed to the confusion by referring to the staff of Aesculapius as the caduceus of Aesculapius and by having a French military publication called *La Caducée*.

In 1917, Colonel McCulloch (the librarian for the surgeon general of the US) discovered in his records a coloured coat of arms prepared for the US medical corps. This emblem depicted the staff of Aesculapius in the left half of the shield, while the right half displayed the US flag. The number of stars on the flag dated its creation to the 1817 founding-date of the US medical corps[40]. He and other historians were unable to understand why the original insignia was ignored and why the error has not been corrected[38,39]. The erroneous medical symbolism used by the US army was copied by many emerging medical organizations with the result that, even today, some continue to regard the caduceus as the proper symbol of medicine. This fallacy has been nurtured intellectually by neologists and some lexicographers who have committed symbolic blasphemy by dubbing the staff of Aesculapius as a medical caduceus. There is no sound historical basis for this etymological error which has been promulgated by some medical organizations and academics as well as the media. Although many American medical historians have hoped that the American army would correct its symbolism, some physicians have grown to love the caduceus. The caduceus' continued association with medicine is based on flimsy and pseudo-historical research. Some evidence exists to consider the caduceus as the logo of Ishtar[41]. Supporters of this view need to reflect on whether or not they would rather practise medicine following the oath of Hippocrates or the code of Hammurabi (king of Babylonia) which punished errors by amputation of the hand.

Asclepius prevails
The staff of Asclepius appears in the coat of arms of most major medical organizations and has almost completely replaced the errant caduceus. The Royal Society of Medicine is an interesting exception. Their coat of arms was not adopted until 122 years after its founding and at that time, in 1927, there was considerable discussion regarding choice of the central emblem and its armorial supporters[42]. Eventually, Sts Cosmas and Damian were chosen to support a tau cross entwined by the brazen serpent of Moses.

The story of the brazen serpent of Moses appears in *Numbers* 21, 6 – 9 of the Holy Bible. Around 1300 BC, Moses was leading the children of Israel across the Sinai desert. They complained about the food and conditions, and ignored God; for this, they were punished with a plague of serpents. Moses sought help from God and was told to make a fiery serpent and erect it on a pole — those who looked on it would live. The remedy worked and the staff and serpent of Moses became a historical forerunner of the staff of Asclepius. In Christian times, God's message was edited such that the staff was depicted as a tau cross. In the Middle Ages, this modified symbol of Moses became a prefiguration of Christ nailed to the cross and the brass serpent became a symbol of healing. The symbolic raising of the serpent and cross was used as a prophylaxis and treatment for the plague epidemics of the 14th to 16th centuries. It was also depicted on the *pesttalers* (plague dollars) of Germany (described in chapter 11). During the Renaissance, the popularity of this symbol and its striking resemblance to the staff of Asclepius aided its modern re-adoption as the symbol of medicine. By serendipity, the Royal Society of Medicine's coat of arms is a reminder of this little-known fact, and to the uninitiated the tau cross and serpent remain suggestive of the staff of Asclepius (Figure 75).

Happily, the ancient god of medicine also enjoys a physical presence inside the Royal Society of Medicine where a replica statue stands in a niche; there is also a second century copy of an ancient head of Asclepius in the members' lounge. Outside, two bronze lamps resembling the serpent-entwined altar lamps of Epidaurus flank its portals (Figure 80). Most of the Society's 17,000 members from

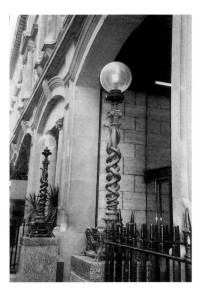

Figure 80 Serpent-entwined lamps outside the Royal Society of Medicine, London (Photo GDH). Compare with the altar lamps at Pergamum (Figure 27)

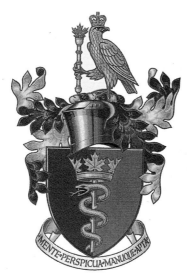

Figure 81   The staff of Asclepius is the central symbol of the coat of arms of the Royal College of Physicians and Surgeons of Canada (Courtesy Royal College of Physicians and Surgeons of Canada, Ottawa, ON, Canada). The staff is stout and knobby, and the serpent appears ferocious rather than the friendly, domesticated *Elaphe longissima* used in the temples

Britain and abroad belong to medical associations whose insignia include the staff and serpent of Asclepius (Figure 81). The Royal Society of Medicine has created an academic union of the rival icons from medical history.

Summary

The art and science of medical care developed by the followers of Asclepius were the foundations on which 20th century medical practice has developed. The staff of Asclepius remains a symbolic link between the clinical and ethical practices of Hippocratic physicians and present-day medical progress. It has witnessed the success of modern medicine performing the miracles sought from Asclepius, and the diverse disciplines associated with healthcare will take the staff and serpent symbol into its fourth millennium.

**PIO
VSLLM
DURNOVARIAE
MM**

Notes and references

1. Barns JWB. *BMJ* 1964; **2**: 567.
2. Jones WHS. *Hippocrates* Vol 1. Loeb Classical Library. Massachusetts: Harvard University Press, 1984.
3. Nutton V. What's in an oath? *J R Coll Physicians Lond* 1995; **29**(6): 518–24.
4. Edelstein L. The Hippocratic oath: text, translation and interpretation. *Bull Hist Med* 1943; **1**(suppl 5): 1–64. © The Johns Hopkins University Press. Text and apparatus criticus taken from Heiberg IL, ed. *Hippocratic opera, corpus medicorum graecorum 1*, 1927: 4–5.
5. The letter itself belongs in the least acceptable category of reliable Hippocratic material but its importance is the reference to the ceremony. The letter also shows Hippocrates' prestige as the people of Abdera in northern Greece (Thrace) are requesting him to consult on the mental state of the city's famous philosopher, Democritus. Hippocrates took the long trip and ended up prescribing hellebore to purge a minor mental condition.
6. Code of Ethics of the Canadian Medical Association. *Can Med Assoc J*, Oct 15 1996: 155.
7. Kenny PN. The CMA Code of Ethics: more room for reflection. *Can Med Assoc J*, Oct 15 1996: 155.
8. Defining the physician's duty to inform. Consensus statement Ontario's expert panel on duty to inform. *Can Med Assoc J* June 2 1998: 158.
9. Press release. *BMA updates Hippocratic oath*. London: British Medical Association, March 27 1997.
10. For Greek text see: Goold GP, ed. *Hippocrates vol 1*. Loeb Classical Library. Massachusetts: Harvard University Press; reprinted 1984.
11. For Greek text see: Goold GP, ed. *Epidemics vol 1*. Loeb Classical Library. Massachusetts: Harvard University Press; reprinted 1984.
12. For Greek text see: Goold GP, ed. *Aphorisms* I, 1, *vol 4*. Loeb Classical Library. Massachusetts: Harvard University Press; reprinted 1984.
13. For Greek text see: Goold GP, ed. *Law* IV, *vol 2*. Loeb Classical Library. Massachusetts: Harvard University Press; reprinted 1984.
14. For Greek text see: Goold GP, ed. *Aphorisms* I, *vol 4*. Loeb Classical Library. Massachusetts: Harvard University Press; reprinted 1984.
15. Peterson MC, Holbrook JH, Hales DV *et al.* Contributions of the history, physical examination and laboratory investigation in making medical diagnoses. *West J Med* 1992; **156**: 163–5.
16. Bordage B. Where are the history and physical? *Can Med Assoc J*, May 15 1995: 152.
17. Chadwick J, Mann WN. *The medical works of Hippocrates*. Oxford: Blackwell Scientific Publications, 1950.
18. Glaxo Wellcome is one of the world's largest pharmaceutical companies.
19. Houston C, Stuart. Scurvy and Canadian exploration. *Can Bull Hist Med* 1990; **7**: 161–7. There was no pharmacist on this expedition and the exact tree used has been debated. Recent investigations have identified the tree as the Eastern White Cedar (*Thuga occidentalis*).
20. Louis Hébert was a brother in a religious order that was related to the Order of St John of God located on Tiber island.
21. Bender GA. *Great moments in pharmacy*. Detroit: Northwood Institute Press, 1966.
22. Polunin M, Robbins C. *The natural pharmacy*. Vancouver: Raincoast Books, 1993.
23. Hart GD. Ancient coins and medicine. *Can Med Assoc J* 94, pp. 77–89, Jan.8, 1966.

24. Vincaleucoblastine (editorial). *Can Med Assoc J* 85; pp. 610–611, 1961.
25. Noble RL, Beer CT, Cutts JH. *Ann New York Acad Sci* 1958; **76**: 882.
26. The process continues and the most recent significant discovery has been the presence of a broad-spectrum antibiotic in the stomach of the dogfish shark. This antibiotic has been isolated and is now produced synthetically in the laboratory by genetic engineering. Glousiusz J. The secret healing power of sharks. *Discovery* Jan 1994: 86.
27. Hamilton JS. Scribonius Largus on the medical profession. *Bull Hist Med* 1986; **60**: 209–16.
28. *Report of the board of science and education on alternative therapy.* London: British Medical Association, 1986.
29. Hodges RD, Scofield AM. Is spiritual healing a valid and effective therapy? *J R Soc Med* 1995; **88**: 203–7.
30. Such an explanation is hard to accept, but current scientific methods cannot explain the migratory habits of birds!
31. The College of Physicians and Surgeons of Ontario consider reassuring gestures, that involve any form of touch, liable to be interpreted as a latent form of sexual harassment.
32. There is a third century BC representation of the Egyptian god, Thoth, holding a staff entwined by a single serpent. There is nothing else to associate the origin of the Asclepian staff with Egypt, apart from a hint that the concept of Asclepian temple medicine might have been brought to Greece by Greek traders familiar with Egyptian customs.
33. Bartlow RM. The origin of the caduceus. *Aesculapius* 1971; **1**: 8–10.
34. Friedlander WJ. *The golden wand of medicine — a history of the caduceus symbol in medicine.* New York: Greenwood Press, 1992.
35. Schouten J. *The rod and serpent of Asklepios.* New York: Elsevier Publishing Company, 1967.
36. Newman C. Transcript from old portrait catalogue of the Royal College of Physicians. [Personal communication.]
37. The Holbein portrait of William Harvey portrayed a caduceus but did not indicate a medical role as Harvey used it in 1598 when he was studying at Padua. He did not graduate in medicine until four years later and his use at that time either represented his interest in pharmacology and chemistry or was part of his family crest.
38. Bremer JL. The caduceus again. *N Engl J Med* 1958; **258**(7): 334–6.
39. Laughlin VC. The Aesculapian staff and the caduceus as medical symbols. *J Int Col Surgeons* 1962; **37**(4).
40. McCulloch CC Jr. Coat of arms of the medical corps. *Military Surgery* 1917; **41**: 137.
41. Michael R. Hermes? Apollo? Ningishzida? *Dracunculus?* ... *Dracunculus??* [Letter.] *JAMA* 1989; **262**(13): 1771.
42. Sir Donald Harrison, president of the Royal Society of Medicine 1994–6, reviewed the herb All-heal which was portrayed in the Society's crest of the coat of arms. His research led to the conclusion that the botanical illustration was not accurate but that the herb depicted was *Stachys officinalis*, the hedge nettle or betony. *RSM News Report* Session 1995/96; Issue 5. This plant was called Vetticona by the Romans and later became Betonica and hence betony. Musa introduced it to Rome and wrote a treatise containing 47 prescriptions for its use in a variety of ailments. This may have resulted in it also being called All-heal. The flowering stems contain tannins, bitters, essential oils and alkaloids; they were dispensed as a dry powder or an infusion to treat diarrhoea, inflammations and neuralgia.

Further reading

Akerman JY. *Coins of Romans relating to Britain.* London: John Russel Small, 1844.

Aldington, Richard, Ames Delano (Translators). *Larousse encyclopaedia of mythology.* London: Batchworth Press Ltd, 1959.

A catalogue of the Greek coins in the British Museum. London: British Museum:

   Vol 1. Italy. Poole RS, 1873.

   Vol 2. Sicily. Poole RS, 1876.

   Vol 3. Thrace. Head BB and Gardner P, 1877.

   Vol 4. The Seleucid Kings of Syria. Gardner P, 1878.

   Vol 5. Macedonia. Head BV and Gardner P, 1879.

   Vol 6. The Ptolemies. Kings of Egypt. Poole RS, 1883.

   Vol 7. Thessaly to Aetolia. Gardner P, 1883.

   Vol 8. Central Greece. Head BV, 1884.

   Vol 9. Crete and Aegean Islands. Wroth W, 1886.

   Vol 10. Peloponnesus (excluding Corinth). Gardner P, 1887.

   Vol 11. Attica, Megaris, Aegina. Head BB, 1888.

   Vol 12. Corinth and Colonies of Corinth. Head BV, 1884.

   Vol 13. Pontus, Paphlagonia, Bithynia, Bosphorus. Wroth W, 1889.

   Vol 14. Ionia. Head BV, 1892.

   Vol 15. Mysia. Wroth W, 1892.

   Vol 16. Alexandria and the Nomes. Poole RS, 1892.

   Vol 17. Troas, Aeolis, Lesbos. Wroth W, 1894.

   Vol 18. Caria and Islands. Head BV, 1897.

   Vol 19. Lycia, Pamphylia and Pisidia. Hill GF, 1897.

   Vol 20. Galatia, Cappadocia, Syria. Wroth W, 1899.

   Vol 21. Lycaonia, Isauria, Sicilia. Hill GF, 1900.

   Vol 22. Lydia. Hill GF, 1901.

   Vol 23. Parthia. Wroth W, 1903.

Vol 24. Cyprus. Hill GF, 1904.

Vol 25. Phrygia. Head BV, 1906.

Vol 26. Phoenicia. Hill GF, 1910.

Vol 27. Palestine (Galilee, Samaria and Judea). Hill GF, 1914.

Vol 28. Arabia, Mesopotamia, Persia, (Nabatea, Arabia, Provincia, S Arabia, Mesopotamia, Babylon, Assyria, Persia, Alexandrian Empire of the East, Persia, Elymais and Characene), Hill GF, 1922.

Vol 29. Cyrenaica. Robinson ESG, 1927.

Bury JB. *A history of the Roman empire from its foundation to the death of Marcus Aurelius* (27 BC–180 AD). 5th edn. London: John Murray, 1908.

Cary M. *History of Rome*. 2nd edn. London: MacMillan & Co Ltd, 1962.

Collingwood RG, Wright RP. *The Roman inscriptions of Britain (Inscriptions on Stone)*. Oxford: Clarendon Press, 1965.

Cunliffe B. *The Celtic world*. New York, San Francisco and St Louis: McGraw-Hill Book Company, 1979.

Encyclopaedia Britannica: Julian, 1946; **13**: 178.

Encyclopaedia Britannica: The inquisition, 1946; **12**: 377–83.

Green M. *The Gods of the Celts*. Gloucester: Alan Sutton, 1986.

Hammond NGL. *Atlas of the Greek and Roman world in antiquity*. New Jersey: Noyes Press, 1981.

Hassall MWC, Tomlin RSO. *Roman Britain in 1946*. II Inscriptions B. Instrumentum Domesticum, 426–49.

Hill PV, Kent JPC, Carson RAG. *Late Roman bronze coinage AD 324–489*. London: Spink and Sons Ltd, 1960.

Goold GP, ed. *Hippocrates. Vols I, II, IV*. Translated by Jones WHJ. Loeb Classical Library. Massachusetts: Harvard University Press and London: William Heinemann Ltd. Reprinted vol I 1984, vol II 1992, vol IV 1992.

Goold GP, ed. *Hippocrates. Vols V & VI*. Translated by Potter P. Loeb Classic Library. Massachusetts: Harvard University Press and London: William Heinemann Ltd, 1988.

Hoadley M. *The Roman herbal*. Newcastle-upon-Tyne: Frank Graham, 1991.

Horsley J. *Britannia Romana*. Newcastle-upon-Tyne: Frank Graham, 1974.

Jackson R. *Doctors and diseases in the Roman empire*. London: British Museum Publications, 1988.

Kerenyi C. *Asklepios*. New York: Pantheon Books Inc, 1959.

King A. *Roman Gaul and Germany*. London: British Museum Publications, 1990.

Lyons AS, Petrucelli RJ. *Medicine: an illustrated history*. New York: Harry N Abrams Inc, 1978.

MacCana P. *Celtic mythology*. London: The Hamlyn Publishing Group, 1970.

Margotta R. *An illustrated history of medicine*. London: The Hamlyn Publishing Group, 1968.

Mattingley H. *Coins of the Roman empire in the British Museum*. London: Trustees of the British Museum:

  Vol I: Augustus to Vitellius, 1922.

  Vol II: Vespasian to Domitian, 1930.

  Vol III: Nerva to Hadrian, 1936.

  Vol IV: Antoninus Pius to Commodus, 1940.

  Vol V: Pertinax to Elagabalus, 1950.

  Vol VI: Severus Alexander to Balbinus & Pupienus, Carson, RAG, reprinted 1976.

Graf F. *Oxford classical dictionary*. 3rd edn. Oxford: Oxford University Press, 1996.

Rodwell W, ed. *Temples, churches and religions in Roman Britain*. BAR 1980; 77(1).

Roman Imperial Coinage:

  Vol V: Part I, Mattingly H, Sydenham EA.

  Vol V: Part II, Webb PH, Probus to Amandus. London: Spink & Sons Ltd, 1933.

  Vol VI: Carson RAG & Sutherland CHV, Diocletian's reform to the death of Maximinus. London: Spink & Sons Ltd, 1967.

  Vol VII: Bruun PM. Constantine and Licinius. London: Spink & Sons Ltd, 1966.

  Vol VIII: Sutherland CHV, Carson RAG, Kent JBC. The Family of Constantine 337–64 AD. London: Spink & Sons Ltd, 1981.

  Vol IX: Pearce JWE. Valentinian I to Theodosius I. London: Spink & Sons Ltd, 1951.

Schouten J. *The rod and serpent of Asklepios*. New York: Elsevier Publishing Company, 1967.

Shulman. The Hans MF Gallery. *Coins of the Roman World*, (Catalogue). New York: Thomas Ollive Mabbott Collection Parts I and II 1969 (Hans Holzer, Editor).

Spencer WG. *Celsus, de Medicina; vol I–IV*. Massachusetts: Harvard University Press, 1960.

Stoneman R, Wallace R. *Classical Association wall map. Ancient Greece and the Aegean*. London: Routledge.

Storer HR. *Medicina in Nummis*. Massachusetts: Wright and Potter Printing, 1931.

Thompson CH. *The Thompson chain-reference Bible*. BB Kirkbride Bible Co Inc,

Indianapolis, Indiana and Zondervan Bible Publishers, Grand Rapids, Michigan. Third Printing 1984.

Watts D. *Christians and pagans in Roman Britain*. London: Routledge, 1991.

Webster G. *The British Celts and their gods under Rome*. London: BT Batsford Ltd, 1986.

Gove PB, ed. *Webster's third new international dictionary (unabridged)*. Springfield, Massachusetts: G&C Merriam Co, 1961.

Webster's biographical dictionary. Springfield, Massachusetts: G&C Merriam Co, 1962.

Webster's geographical dictionary. Springfield, Massachusetts: G&C Merriam Company, 1963.

Webster's medical desk dictionary. Springfield, Massachusetts: Merriam-Webster Inc.

Woodward A. *Shrines and sacrifice*. London: BT Batsford Ltd/English Heritage, 1992.

Appendix 1

Numismatic notes: coin illustrations

The photographs show varying degrees of magnification.

Metal type is indicated by: (AU) = gold; (AR) = silver; (AE) = bronze. (Please note that 'AR' is the abbreviation for the Latin argentum (silver).)

The symbol for the British Museum Catalogue (BMC) metal type is followed by bracketed numbers — these indicate the diameter of the coin in decimals of an inch and/or its weight in grains (1 grain = 0.0648 grams). The BMC volumes have a conversion table for English inches into millimetres and the relative weight of English grains and French grammes. These tables are, themselves, historical documents!

Figure 1

a) BMC 10, Peloponnesus, Epidaurus, 329–240 BC, Drachm (AR 0.75, 61.0) P.156 #7

b) CNG XXIII #227 Oct 92

c) BMC 8, Central Greece, Phocis, Delphi. Obverse Faustina Senior, (AE 0.95) #34. Coin inscribed 'PYTHIA', which was the name of the priestess who sat at the entrance of the cave at Delphi. This inscription appears on coins from: Cibyra and Hieropolis in Phyrgia (BMC, 25); Thyatira and Tralles in Lydia (BMC, 22); Ancyra in Galatia (BMC 20); Termessus major in Pisidia (BMC 19); Emesa in Syria (BMC 20); Phocidis and Delphi in the Peloponnesus (BMC 10); Perinthus and Philippolis in Thrace (BMC 3) and Aphrodisias in Caria (BMC 18)

Figure 3

a) Minted by Hadrian in the name of Sabina. BMC 15, Mysia, Pergamum (AE 0.8) P.144 #274

b) BMC 13, Bithynia (AE 0.88) # 210

c) BMC 12, Colony of Corinth, Acharnania, Leucas (AR 0.85, 131.3) #61

The Corinthian Athena was depicted as a younger and less stern goddess than the portrait type of Athens and the Roman depictions of Minerva. The small figure on the left is Hermes with Caduceus and with his left leg raised fixing his sandal or ? indicating his ancillary role with the lower extremity

d) Macedonia, Neapolis, fifth to fourth century BC, AR Hemidrachm (1.79 gm), SNG, ANS 456

f) BMC 18, Caria, Attuda (AE 0.95) P.65 # 20

Figure 4

a) BMC 15, Mysia, Pergamum (133 BC–Augustus) (AE 0.7) P. 129 #158

b) BMC 18, Caria, Cos (166–88 BC) (AR 0.55) P.207 #136

Figure 6

a) BMC 10, Peloponnesus, Epidaurus, 323–240 BC, Drachm (AR 0.75, 61.0) P.156 #7

b) BMC 7, Thessaly to Aetolia, Larissa (AR 0.5), 450–400 BC, P.28 #44

Figure 7 BMC 3, Thrace, 244 AD minted by Philippus Senior (AE 1.6) #8

Figure 8

a) BMC 17 ,Troas, Aeolis, Lesbos. Myrina (AR 1.25) (first to second century BC) #2

b) BMC 17, Myrina (first to second century BC) (AR 1.35) #1

c) BMC 17, Myrina (first to second century BC) (AR 1.3) #1

Figure 9

a) Bruttium, Caulonia, AR Nomos, c525–480 BC. CNG XVIII, 1993 # 20

b) Bruttium, Croton, AR Stater, 510 BC. CNG Vol 3 1992 # 21

c) Myrina, Aeolis, AR tetradrachm, BC165. CNG XXVII 1993 # 578

Figure 10 RIC, Mattingly & Sydenham, Vol IV, Part 1 Caracalla on obverse, Mint of Rome, (AU) aureus, 207 AD, (picture actual size ×2) #99

Figure 12

a) BMC 15, Mysia, Pergamum (133 BC–Augustus) (AE 0.7) P.129 #158

b) BMC 10, Peloponnesus, Epidaurus, (third to fourth century BC) (AE 0.7) P.157 #11

Figure 13

a) Sestertius of Maximinus I, RIC, IV, Part 2, 236–8 AD (AE 1.2) #35

b) BMC 15, Mysia, Pergamum, L.Verus (161–9 AD) (AE 1.6) P.147 #291

Figure 16 BMC 15, Mysia, Perperene (AE 0.6) P.169 #7

Figure 18 Coin of Maximinus I (235–8 AD) from Tarsus (Cilicia) (AE 1.44)

Figure 20 Hippocrates on obverse and the staff of Asclepius on the reverse. BMC listed the date as first century BC to Augustus but recent research has shown that the coin belongs to the second century AD when Cos was given a degree of numismatic autonomy. BMC 18, Caria, Cos (AE 0.55) P.216 #216

Figure 21 BMC 15, Mysia, Pergamum, Caracalla on the obverse (AE 1.75) P.156 #326

Figure 24

a) Cos (88–50 BC); Asclepius on the obverse and the staff of Asclepius on the reverse

BMC 18, Caria Cos (AE 0.9) P.211 #178

Figure 27 BMC 15, Mysia, Pergamum (AE 1.0) P.147 #290

Figure 28

a) BMC 13, Pontus, Paphlagonia, Bithynia and Bosphorus Abonoteichus (AE 1.16) P.83 #1

b) BMC 26, Phoenicia, Berytus (AE 1.0) #219

c) BMC 16, Alexandria and the Nomes, Claudius, Egypt, (AE 1.0) #101

Figure 30 BMC 10, Peloponnesus, Epidaurus. Asclepius on the obverse. 323–240 BC (AE 0.55) P.158 #25

Figure 31

a) The obverse of this coin type showed either Asclepius or Apollo 323–240 BC BMC 10, Peloponnesus, Epidaurus (AE 0.55) P.158 #24 & 23

b) BMC 10, Peloponnesus, Epidaurus 323–240 BC (AE 0.6) P.157 #12

Figure 33 BMC 16, Alexandria and the Nomes, Alexandria. Hadrianic, AE, P.103 #885

Figure 35

a) BMC 15, Mysia, Pergamum, Commodus (AE 1.4) P.148 #295

b) BMC 15, Mysia, Pergamum, Caracalla (AE 1.8) P.156 #327

c) BMC 15, Mysia, Pergamum, Caracalla (AE 1.75) P.155 #324

d) BMC 15, Mysia, Pergamum, Commodus (AE 0.8) P.149 #302

Figure 36

a) BMC 15, Mysia, Pergamum (211–130 BC) (AE 0.6) P.122 #84

b) BMC 15, Mysia, Pergamum inscribed 'Gymnasiarch' (AE 0.75) P.138 #239

Figure 48 BMC 15, Mysia, Pergamum (AE 1.6) P.148 #292

Figure 50 Reverse of a commemorative medallion struck 140–3 AD in advance of the celebrations commemorating the 900th anniversary of Rome in 147 AD. Obverse shows Antoninus Pius (138–61 AD) (AE 1.48, 42.5) C 2, P.271 #17 and CNG 50, June 99 #334

Figure 51 83 BC Senator Lucius Rubrius Dossenus BAB II, P.408 #6

Figure 56 Denarius 54 BC Man Acilius Glabrio (AR 0.72), S/R/S/C I Acilia #8

Figure 57 Claudius 44 AD, AU (7.84 gm) RIC I, 33

Figure 58 BMC 18, Caria, Cos, second century AD. Xenophon on obverse. (AE 0.85 & 0.75) P.215 #211 & 216. Two types with reverse of 0.85 depicting Hygieia and reverse of 0.75 depicting staff of Asclepius. See Figure 20

Figure 65 Denarius of Caracalla (AR 0.8) C 302

Figure 67

a) BMC 7, Thessaly to Aetolia, Pherae, 450–400 BC (AR 0 .7) P.46 #4

b) BMC 29, Cyrenaica, 308–277 BC (AR 0.7), Plate 22, #27B

Figure 70

a) Constantine 310–3 AD, Trier mint RIC VI #890

b) Lyons mint, AE 2 C 511

Figure 71 Vetranio, 350 AD, Siscia mint, AE Centenionalis Sear 4042

Figure 72 Magnentius, 351–2 AD, Amiens mint, inscribed 'Salus DD NN Aug et Caes'. Chi rho with α and ω. HKC Part 2 #24

Figure 73

Constantine, Constantinople mint (326–30 AD)

a) HKC Part I # 978

b) Wroxeter/Durham. Casey PJ, R Brickstock cat no 1632, (13.5 mm 1.7 g)

Appendix 2

Abbreviations

BAB Babelon E. *Description historique et chronoloogique des Monnaies de la Republique Romaine.* Vols 1 & 2. Paris, 1885–6

BAR *British Archaeology Reports*

BMC *Catalogues of Greek coins* in the British Museum, 1873–1927. Photographs reproduced with permission from the Trustees of the British Museum © Copyright The British Museum

BMJ *British Medical Journal*

BHM *Bulletin of the History of Medicine*

C Cohen H. *Déscription historique des monnaies frappées sous L'Empire Romain, communément appelées Medailles Impériales.* 2nd edn. 1880.

CBHM *Canadian Bulletin of the History of Medicine*

CMA Canadian Medical Association

CMAJ *Canadian Medical Association Journal*

CNG Classic Numismatic Group Inc, Lancaster, Pennsylvania, US and London, England

CNR *Classical Numismatic Review*, incorporating the *Seaby Coin and Medal Bulletin*, Lancaster, Pennsylvania and London, England

CRE Coins of the Roman empire in the British Museum

Enc B *Encyclopaedia Britannica*

FR Further reading

GDH Gerald D Hart

HKC Hill PV, Kent JPC, Carson RAG. *Late Roman bronze coinage 324–489 AD.* London: Spink and Sons Ltd, 1960

HMSO Her Majesty's Stationery Office

JAMA *Journal of the American Medical Association*

JRSM *Journal of the Royal Society of Medicine*

M&W Photo by Peter Milligan and/or Ian Whan from the Department of Photography, Toronto East General Hospital

NC The Numismatic Chronicle, *Journal of the Royal Numismatic Society*, London

NEJM *New England Journal of Medicine*

PSAS *Proceedings of the Society of Antiquaries of Scotland*

RAC *Revue Archéologique du centre de la France*

RIB Collingwood RG, Wright RP. *Roman inscriptions in Britain*. Oxford, 1965

RIC *Roman Imperial Coinage*, London 1923–33

SNG ANS *Sylloge Nummorum Graecorum, American Numismatic Society*, New York 1969

SRSC I Seaby HA. *Roman silver coins*, volume 1 (Republic to Augustus). 3rd edn. London: Seaby, 1978

SRCS II Seaby HA. *Roman silver coins*, volume 1 (Tiberius to Commodus). 3rd edn. London: Seaby, 1979

Appendix 3

Table 2 368 Asclepian temple sites identified by Walton from coins, archaeology and epigraphy[1]

Location	Temple site
THESSALY:	Atarax*, Kierion*, Krannon, Lakereia, Larissa*, Phlanna, Pherai, Pharsalos, Tricca*, Iolkos
MAGNESIA:	Magnesia*
EPEIROS:	Ambrakia, Nikopolis*
KORKYRA:	Korkyra*
AKARNANIA:	Anaktorion
LOKRIS OZOLIS:	Amphissa, Naupaktos
PHOKIS:	Drymaia, Elateia, Panopeus, Stiris, Tithorea
BOETIA:	Hyettos, Orchomenos, Tanagra, Thespiai, Thisbe
ATTICA:	Acharnai, Athens × 4*, Peiraeus
MEGARIS:	Megara*, Pagai*
KORINTHOS:	Kenchreiai, Korinthos*, Sikyon*, Titane
PHLIASIA:	Phlious*
ARGOLIS:	Argos*, Asine*, Epidauros*, Hermione, Kleone*, Lessa, Troizen*
ACHAIA:	Aigion*, Aigeira*, Araxos, Kyros, Olenos, Patrai*, Pellene*
ARKADIA:	Aliphera, Gortys, Heraia, Kaphyai*, Kaus, Kleitor*, Mantineia*, Megalopolis, Orchomenos*, Phigalea*, Tegea, Thelpusa
ELIS:	Kyllene, Olympia, Forty stadia from ridge of Sauros was a Temple
ZAKYNTHOS:	Zakynthos*
MESSENIA:	Abia, Asine*, Gerenia, Korone, Kyparissiaii*, Messene*, Pylos*, Thuria*
LAKONIA:	Asopos × 2, Boiai*, Brasiai, Epidauros Limera × 2, Gytheion*, Helos, Hypsoi, Kyphanta, Las × 2*, Leuktra, Pallana, Sparta × 2*, Therai
MOESIA:	Anchialos*, Dionysopolis*, Marcianopolis*, Nikopolis*, Tomi*
NORTH of BLACK SEA:	Hagion, Pantikapaion*
DALMATIA:	Narona, Salona
PANNONIA INFERIOR:	Aquincum, Campona, Intercisa, Salva
PANNONIA SUPERIOR:	Julia Emona
NORICUM:	Virinum
DACIA:	Also-Ilosva, Ampelum, Alba Julia, Carlsburg, Cibinium, Galt, Mehadia, Ulpia Trajana
CHERSONESOS:	Chersonesos*
THRACE:	Ainos*, Bizye*, Byzantium*, Deultum*, Hadrianopolis*, Maroneia*, Mesembria*, Odessos*, Pantalia*, Perinthos*, Philippopolis*, Plotinopolis*, Serdika*, Topiros*, Trajanopolis*, Hephaistia*
MACEDONIA:	Amphipolis, Dium*, Pera
PONTUS:	Amasea*, Amasos*, Kerasos*
PAPHYLAGONIA:	Abonoteichos*, Neoclaudiopolis*
BITHYNIA:	Amastris*, Bithynium*, Caesareia-Germanica*, Chalkedon, Hadrianus*, Hadrianothera*, Heraklea*, Juliopolis*, Kios*, Nikaia*, Nicomedia*, Prusa (ad Hypium)*, Prusa (ad Olympum)*, Tium*
TROAS:	Abydos*, Alexandria Troas, Kelainai
AEOLIS:	Aigai*, Assos*, Elaia*, Gargara*, Kame*, Kyme*, Neotichos*, Temnos*
LESBOS:	Mytilene*
MYSIA:	Adramytion*, Antandros*, Apollonia*, Attaia*, Germe*, Kamena*, Kyzikos*, Parion*, Pergamum*, Pionia*, Pitane*, Perperene*, Poimamenos*, Porselene*, Stratonikeia (ad Caicum)*, Thebe*

(Continued)

Table 2   (*continued*)

Location	Temple site
IONIA:	Apollonia*, Ephesos*, Klazomenai*, Kolophon*, Magnesia*, Miletos*, Phokaia, Smyrna*, Teos*
LYDIA:	Akrasos*, Apollonis*, Attalia*, Daldis*, Dioshieron*, Gordus-Julia*, Herakleia*, Hermokapelia*, Hypaipa*, Hyrkania*, Kilbiani*, Maionia*, Magnesia *, Nakrasa *, Philadelphia*, Saittenai*, Thyateira × 2*
KARIA:	Antiochia*, Apollonia*, Baiaca, Bargasa*, Bargylia*, Chersonesos*, Euippe*, Halikarnassos*, Knidos*, Mylasa, Peraia, Pharasa*, Stratonikeia*, Trapezopolis*
DORIAN ISLANDS:	Astypalaia*, Chalke, Karpathos, Kasos, Kos × 3*, Crete (Lebena)*, Priansos*, Rhodos, Thera
PHRYGIA:	Aizanis*, Akmonia*, Ankyra*, Attalia*, Attuda*, Bruzas*, Dionysopolis*, Dokimaion*, Eukarpia*, Grimenothyrae*, Hierapolis*, Hieropolis*, Kadi*, Kibyra*, Kidyessos*, Kolossai*, Kotiaion*, Lampsakos, Laodikeia*, Midaion*, Nakolea*, Otrus*, Peltai*, Prymnessos*, Sala*, Siblia*, Stektorion*, Synaos*, Synnada*, Themisonion*, Tiberopolis*, Tripolis*
PISIDIA:	Antiochia*, Ariassos*, Lyrbe*, Sagallos*, Selge*
LYKIA:	Rhodiopolis
PAMPHYLIA:	Attalia*
LYKAONIA:	Parlais*
KILIKIA:	Aigai*, Argos*, Irenopolis*, Kolybrassos*, Lyrbe*, Soli, Syedra*, Tarsos*
GALATIA:	Ankyra*, Pessisus*, Sebaste*, Tanion*
KAPADOKIA:	Kataonia, Tyana*
ISLANDS of the AEGEAN:	Aigina, Amorgos*, Anchiale*, Anaphe, Delos, Klaros, Kythera, Melos, Paros, Pordoselene, Samos, Syros
PHOENICIA:	Grove between Berytos and Sidon, Tyre*
MEDIA:	Ekbatana
SAMARIA:	Caesarea*
JUDEA:	Ascalon
EGYPT:	Alexandria*, Memphis, Philis, Ptolemais
MAURETANIA:	Caesarea
NUMIDIA:	Calama, Lambaesis, Ulpia Marciana Trajana
AFRICA (in general):	Carthage, Chisidio, Hamman Ellif, Kyrene, Balagrai, Municipium Thibica, Thibursicum, Thignica
ITALY:	Aeclanum, Amiternum, Atina, Asculum, Auximum, Bononia, Croton, Etruria*, Grotta Ferrata, Pompeii, Praeneste, Puteoli, Rhegium*, Rome × 2*, Tarentum, Tegianum
SICILY:	Agrigentum*, Menaenum*, Messana, Selinus*, Syracuse*, Paulus Gerreus
SARDINIA:	Cerales
GALLIA CISALPINA:	Aquileia, Bellunum, Libactium, Pola, Taurini
GALLIA NARBONENSIS:	Augustum, Gratianopolis, Nemausus, Reii
HISPANIA:	Bracera Augusta, Caldas de Vizella, Carthago Nova, Merobriga, Nescania, Olisipo, Saguntum, Valentia
ENGLAND:	Ellenborough (Maryport), Lancaster (Lanchester), Chester

Ellenborough (Alauna) is now known as Maryport; Lancaster (Longovicium) is Lanchester, Chester (Deva)

Thrace listing of Pantalia may represent Pataulia in Thrace

*= coins portraying Asclepius, Hygieia or Telesphorus were minted there

×2= two temple sites known; ×4 = four temple sites known

Table 3   165 Asclepian temple sites identified solely by coins[1]

Location	Site
THESSALY	Atrax, Kieron, Larissa
THRACE	Ainos, Bizye, Byzantium, Deultum, Maroneia, Mesembra, Pantalia (?Pataulia), Perinthos, Philippopolis, Plotinopolis, Serdica, Topiros, Trajanopolis, Hephaistia
MACEDONIA	Dium
ZAKYNTHOS	Zakynthos
MESSENIA	Abia, Pylos, Thuria
MAGNESIA	Homolian
EPEIROS	Nikopolis
MEGARIS	Pagai
ARGOLIS	Asine, Hermione
ACHAIA	Pellene
ARKADIA	Orchomenos, Phigalea
PAPHLAGONIA	Neoclaudiopolis
BITHYNIA	Amastris, Bithynium, Caesareia-Germanica, Hadrianus Hadrianothera, Heraklea, Juliopolis, Kios, Nikaia, Nikomedia, Prusa (ad Hyphium), Prusa (ad Olympium), Tium, Orchomenos
TROAS	Abydos
AEOLIS	Aigai, Assos, Gargara, Kame, Kyme, Neontichos, Temnos
MOESIA	Anchialos, Dionysopolis, Marcinopolis, Nikopolis, Tomi
MYSIA	Adramytion, Antandros, Apollonia, Attaia, Germe, Kamena, Kyzikos, Parion, Pionia, Pitane, Perperene, Porselene, Stratonikeia, Thebe
IONIA	Apollonia, Ephesos, Klazomenai, Kolophon, Magnesia, Phokaia
CHERSONESOS	Chersonesos
PONTUS	Amasea, Amasos, Kerasos
LYDIA	Akrasos, Apollonis, Attalia, Daldis, Dioshieron, Gordus-Julia, Herakleia, Hermokapleia, Hypaipa, Hyrkania, Kilbiani, Maionia, Magnesia, Nakrasa, Philadelphia, Saittenai
KARIA	Antiochia, Apollonia, Bargasa, Bargylia, Chersonesos, Euippe, Halikarnassos, Mylassa, Pharasa, Trapezopolis
PISIDIA	Antiochia, Araissos, Lyrbe, Sagallos, Selge
ISLANDS OF THE AEGEAN SEA	Amorgos, Anchiale
PAMPHYLIA	Attalia
PHOENICIA	Tyre
PHRYGIA	Aizanis, Akmonia, Ankyra, Attalia, Attuda, Bruzas, Dionysopolis, Dokimaion, Eukarpia, Grimenothyrae (Trajanopolis), Heirapolis, Hieropolis, Kadi, Kibyra, Kidyessos, Kolossai, Kotiaion, Laodikeia, Misaion, Nakolea, Otrus, Peltai, Prymnessos, Sala, Siblia, Stektorion, Synaos, Synnada, Themisonion, Tiberopolis, Tripolis
LYKAONIA	Parlais
SAMARIA	Caesarea
KILIKIA	Argos, Irenopolis, Kolybrassos Lyrbe, Syedra, Tarsus
SICILY	Menaenum, Selinus
ITALY	Etruria, Rhegium
GALATIA	Pessinus, Sebaste, Tanion
KAPPADOKIA	Tyana
DORIAN ISLANDS	Priansos

Index

Information on pages in *italics* is contained only in an illustration or caption